Normal Cell Morphology in Canine and Feline Cytology

Normal Cell Morphology in Canine and Feline Cytology
An Identification Guide

Written and translated by
Lorenzo Ressel

DVM, PhD, FHEA, DiplECVP, MRCVS
RCVS and European Veterinary Specialist in Pathology
Senior Lecturer in Veterinary Pathology
Institute of Veterinary Science
University of Liverpool
Liverpool, UK

WILEY Blackwell

Registered Offices
John Wiley & Sons, Inc., 111 River Street, Hoboken, NJ 07030, USA
John Wiley & Sons Ltd, The Atrium, Southern Gate, Chichester, West Sussex, PO19 8SQ, UK

Editorial Office
9600 Garsington Road, Oxford, OX4 2DQ, UK

For details of our global editorial offices, customer services, and more information about Wiley products visit us at www.wiley.com.

Wiley also publishes its books in a variety of electronic formats and by print-on-demand. Some content that appears in standard print versions of this book may not be available in other formats.

Library of Congress Cataloging-in-Publication Data

Names: Ressel, Lorenzo, 1979– author.
Title: Normal cell morphology in canine and feline cytology : an identification guide /
   written and translated by Lorenzo Ressel.
Other titles: Principi di identificazione morfologica in citologia nel cane e nel gatto. English
Description: Hoboken, NJ : Wiley, 2018. | Translation of: Principi di identificazione morfologica in citologia nel cane
   e nel gatto. 2010. | Includes index. | Description based on print version record and CIP data provided by
   publisher; resource not viewed.
Identifiers: LCCN 2017025396 (print) | LCCN 2017027036 (ebook) | ISBN 9781119278917 (pdf) |
   ISBN 9781119278900 (epub) | ISBN 9781119278894 (pbk.)
Subjects: | MESH: Dog Diseases–pathology | Cat Diseases–pathology | Cytodiagnosis–veterinary | Cells–cytology
Classification: LCC SF 991 (ebook) | LCC SF 991 (print) | NLM SF 991 | DDC 636.7/0896–dc23
LC record available at https://lccn.loc.gov/2017025396

Cover design by Wiley
Cover images: courtesy of Lorenzo Ressel

Set in 10/11 pt Optima LT Std by SPi Global, Pondicherry, India

10 9 8 7 6 5 4 3 2 1

Contents

Foreword

Cytology for students, for clinicians or for diagnosticians? I'm sure this question often crossed the mind of the author, Dr. Lorenzo Ressel (a passionate devotee of the discipline, who I have the honor to call a colleague and friend), when he was thinking about the content, style and recipients of the present book, and hoping this would be the first in a long series.

There is a parallel universe, which belongs to the 'infinitely small', that is hidden and elusive, which is only unraveled by the use of a microscope, and that represents an irresistible call for those who are lucky to consider a passion and a job the very same thing.

Very easy to read, compact, useful and complete, this book sets as its first goal, for the student to draw the morphology of the cells in the mind, as they appear in the reality of that microscopic universe, and therefore to build solid foundations for their quick and secure identification. In the same way, the use of this book is also recommended to the professional cytologist, since it provides the instruments to 'scratch' the mnemonic rusts, which sometimes may compromise the ability to interpret and describe.

I followed the progressive development of this work and appreciated Lorenzo's efforts and commitment in his search for meticulous precision and attention to detail, as well as his enthusiasm during the realization of the book.

I'm sure now the answer to my first question is: 'cytology for those who love cells'.

Carlo Masserdotti
Med Vet, Dipl ECVCP, Brescia (IT)

Introduction

The book you hold in your hands is not a classic text of diagnostic cytology of the dog and cat. The starting point is not the needle and the goal is not the diagnosis, but it continues to 'go in circles' around cells.

Due to this particular feature, it could be considered as something preparatory to diagnostic cytology activity and, predominantly, it has been precisely designed for this purpose: to give a comprehensive but original approach to the study of normal cells for the veterinary student interested in diagnostic veterinary cytology, hoping to fill the gap between the first year courses on cell biology, and final year's clinical pathology rotations. I think, however, this book will also find a place close to the microscope of the novice practising veterinary cytologist, when having 'easy-to-use' information to hand is the key to correct interpretation and diagnosis.

A first chapter, *'Cellular biology and cytological interpretation: the philosophy behind the system'*, discusses the principles of morphological identification, trying to clarify the relationship between shapes, patterns and colours and the associated interpretation of cell origin and behaviour.

The second chapter, *'Distribution of cells in tissues and organs'*, aims at clarifying which cells can typically be sampled from the different tissues and organs. Figures showing the location of different cell types in the context of the histological structures of organs guide the reader to an easy identification.

The third chapter, *'Cytotypes'*, is the heart of the book: different cell types from the various organs and tissues are presented as 'identification sheets', arranged in alphabetical order. The cells' characteristics are systematically described in this chapter.

Chapter 4, *'Cytoarchitectures'*, classifies the different morphologies that groups of cells form (or maintain from the original tissue arrangement) when sampled and subsequently smeared over the slide.

The fifth chapter, *'Background'*, discusses the non-cellular material that may be observed alongside cells, and, in some cases, can be peculiar to a particular cytotype.

The sixth chapter, *'Morphological alterations of cells'*, introduces the different cellular morphological alterations which can be observed in different pathological changes, such as degeneration and disturbances of tissue growth.

At the end of the book, instead of a traditional index, there is a unique *'Visual index'*, in which the cytotypes (previously described in the third chapter) are presented together, to scale, to give the reader a quick, visual identification approach.

Cellular biology and cytological interpretation: the philosophy behind the system

◼ Shape and observation

Aside from the mere pleasure of observation, an activity that is in its own way rather satisfying, the ability to extract information from the object observed is based on the axiom that different shapes and colours (of the object observed) correspond to different information.

This concept is at the heart of diagnostic cytology. The person who observes the cells on the slide (the cytologist) can use the morphological features of the cell observed (shape and colour) to classify it and interpret its characteristic biological behaviour.

◼ Morphology, identity and behaviour

If properly interpreted, the different shapes and colours of a cell can provide information about its metabolism and differentiation. Indeed, specific chromatic features of the cytoplasm may indicate a particular cell's metabolic condition. Moreover, certain visible structures can tell us that a cell is dividing (e.g. the presence of a mitotic figure), or that it is undergoing phagocytosis (e.g. the presence of material within the cytoplasm). There are also morphologies that suggest no immediate functional interpretation. Such morphologies are 'structural' and connected to a specific type of cell (e.g. the polylobed nucleus of *neutrophils*).

It is also true that certain cell types, due to their ability to carry out a highly specialized and predetermined function (differentiation), have 'acquired' certain morphological features that make them unique and recognizable from other cells. Examples are *plasma cells*, which, due to their constant protein synthesis, display an intensely blue cytoplasm, or, *macrophages*, whose vacuole-containing cytoplasm is a distinctive feature, as well as an expression of phagocytosis.

This goes to show how from a plethora of shapes one can understand both the 'type of cell being observed', and, at times, 'what it is doing'.

Normal Cell Morphology in Canine and Feline Cytology: An Identification Guide,
First Edition. Written and translated by Lorenzo Ressel.
© 2018 John Wiley & Sons Ltd. Published 2018 by John Wiley & Sons Ltd.

Identity and interpretation

The observation of cellular morphology allows classification of cells into different 'cytotypes', i.e. it enables the cytologist to classify them into a specific category. In diagnostic cytology, it is common to classify cells into three morphological families: epithelial, mesenchymal and discrete, otherwise known as round cells.

Traditionally, these three morphological groups are defined as follows.

- Epithelial cells – usually large and round or polygonal in shape, with readily identifiable cellular margins. These cells usually form clusters, which are aggregates of cells that establish contact by means of membrane-to-membrane adhesion.
- Mesenchymal cells – usually of medium size, they appear elongated, spindle-shaped or pleomorphic. These cells may form aggregates of cells through interposition of matrix.
- Discrete cells – usually small and round, they do not establish contact with each other.

With some obvious exceptions, this classification system is of great diagnostic value, hence, the above-mentioned terms will be referred to several times throughout this book. Within these categories, subtle differences in shape, size, presence or absence of certain structures, location of the nucleus and other significant areas often allow classification of cells into specific 'cytotypes', in other words a cell that *Homo sapiens* has dignified with a name and surname. For example, the ability to selectively identify various cytotypes is crucial to tests such as differential and absolute cell counts, which often provide valuable diagnostic information.

Behaviour and interpretation

The adaptability of cells to outside stimuli or modifications of the environment (hormones, maturative stimuli, etc.) induces the same cytotype to modulate the specific morphological features (shape and identity) it 'normally' displays as it adapts to a new function. The evaluation of these changes, which are compared to the normal morphology of the cytotype (defined by its shapes and colours), allows a higher level of understanding compared to the more basic cellular identification: the cell's metabolic status. This, in turn, has important repercussions on cytological diagnosis, especially in the field of oncology. The variation of these features within a specified *range* will be considered within the normal limits of the phenotype, but a phenotype that is particularly active or reactive will exhibit morphological features far beyond such limits.

Knowledge and interpretation

Each of the features observed in a cell provides specific information that can help both cytotype identification and functional assessment. These features and their biological significance are discussed here individually, in detail. The combination of more features characterizing different cell types will be dealt with in Chapter 3, Cytotypes. The various morphological features observed have been divided into cellular morphologies, nuclear morphologies, cytoplasmic morphologies and supercellular morphologies (those shapes that are determined by the connections between cells).

■ Cellular morphologies

'Cellular morphology' refers to the set of morphological features (shape and colour) of a cell as a whole. The features considered are:

- size;
- shape;
- nuclear:cytoplasmic ratio;
- presence of certain specialized structures.

Size of cells

The size of cells can vary greatly. It ranges from an erythrocyte 6 or 7 µm in diameter, up to a rhabdomyocyte of several hundred microns. Except for those cells whose size can vary greatly because of their specific activities (for example, macrophages can increase their size due to the accumulation of phagocytosed material), the size of a cell is often a useful tool to identify the cytotype.

Usually, very large cells in normal conditions are actually *syncytia*: several cellular bodies merging into one unique cytotype, which is characterized by the presence of multiple nuclei in the cytoplasm.

Cellular shape

The shape of a cell, determined by its margins, can provide valuable information about its classification. In general, a well-defined and repeatable cellular shape is given by its cytoskeleton, which determines the shape when the cell itself is originally located within the tissue and/or organ of origin. On the contrary, so-called *pleomorphic* cells indicate a more plastic cytotype. They will therefore feature a less rigid morphology, which is not characteristic or indicative of the original tissue. Consequently, when a cell is classified as pleomorphic, it is assumed that, within the cytotype to which it belongs, it will not have a specific and repeatable shape.

There are several cells that, within a given cytotype, maintain a typical morphology. A possible classification by shape would include round, ovoid, columnar, fusiform/spindle, cubic, polygonal, star-shaped and pear-shaped cells (Figure 1).

Nuclear:cytoplasmic (or nucleus to cytoplasm) ratio

The nuclear:cytoplasmic ratio determines how much cellular area is occupied respectively by the nucleus and the cytoplasm. A cell whose nucleus occupies almost the entire cellular area is typically at an immature cellular stage. During maturation, cytoplasmic structures (capable of performing different functions), gain space and tend to equalize such area (1:1 ratio) or exceed it. However, there are cases in which cells considered mature retain a high nuclear:cytoplasmic ratio (for example, mature lymphocytes). This feature has, in physiological terms, a major

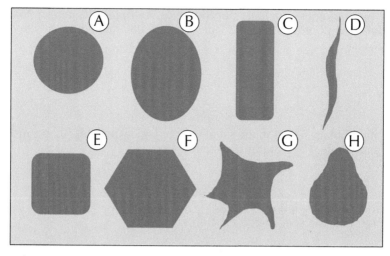

Figure 1 - Schematic representation of the most important cellular morphologies: round (A), ovoid (B), columnar (C), fusiform/spindle (D), cuboidal (E), polygonal (F), star-shaped (G) and pear-shaped (H).

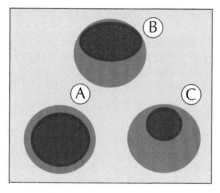

Figure 2 - Schematic representation of the nuclear:cytoplasmic ratio: high (A), equal/intermediate (B) and low (C).

impact on the identification of the cytotype. The implications of this morphological feature with regard to pathological conditions will be dealt with in Chapter 6, Morphological alterations of cells.

The nuclear:cytoplasmic ratio is typically classified as *high* (the nucleus takes up most of the cellular area), *equal/intermediate* (nucleus and cytoplasm occupy approximately the same amount of cellular area) and *low* (the cytoplasm takes up most of the cellular space) (Figure 2). Classifications using numerical values are less typical.

Specialized cellular structures

Some cells have specialized cellular structures, a sign of their specific functional differentiation. Specialized cellular structures are cilia, flagella, microvilli, basal plates, etc. (for more information, see Chapter 3, Cytotypes). These are proof of cellular differentiation, and are thus crucial features for recognizing a cytotype.

■ Nuclear morphologies

'Nuclear morphologies' are those morphological features that affect the nuclear and subnuclear structures (e.g. chromatin and nucleolus). The following characteristics of the nucleus are examined:

- shape;
- position;
- number;
- chromatin patterns;
- nucleolus;
- mitotic figures.

Shape of the nucleus

The nucleus can take different shapes within different cells. This criterion is extremely useful for identification of a particular cytotype. There are nuclear morphologies that are typically associated with a particular cytotype and are not known to be correlated with a particular metabolic state. Generally, they remain unchanged within a cell despite stress of a metabolic nature (e.g. in mature *neutrophils*, the lobulation is generally not lost in cases of stress).

Morphological changes of the nucleus (belonging to a single family of cells) are often a sign of cell maturation. Also in this case, it seems only natural and strategic to classify consecutive and well-identifiable maturation stages by using different names (*cytotypes*) despite merely being different 'ages' of the same cell (e.g. *myeloid* and *erythroid* cells). And that is how we go back to the starting point: the morphology of the nucleus helps to identify cytotypes.

There are several nuclear morphologies: round, oval, spindle-like, kidney-shaped, horseshoe-shaped, indented, bilobed, S-shaped, convoluted and polylobed (Figure 3).

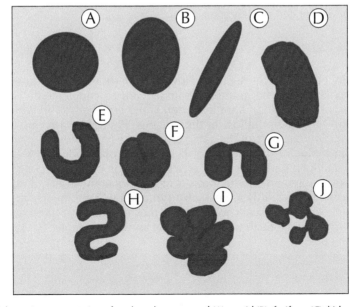

Figure 3 - Schematic representation of nuclear shapes: round (A), ovoid (B), fusiform (C), kidney-shaped (D), horseshoe-shaped (E), indented (F), bilobed (G), S-shaped (H), convoluted (I) and polylobate (J).

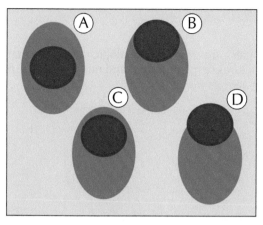

Figure 4 - Schematic representation of the cell nucleus position inside the cell: central (A), paracentral or subterminal (B), peripheral (C) and 'punched out' (D).

Location of the nucleus

The location of the nucleus is another strong indicator when determining a cytotype. The reason why the nucleus is located nearer one of the margins of the cell, and not in the centre, has to do with the fact that the cell has a so-called 'functional polarity', which leads it to amass its cytoplasmic structures on one side, resulting in the formation of a 'pole'.

The shift of the nucleus to the periphery of the cell, can by either due to a constituent cytoplasmic structure increasing in size (rough endoplasmic reticulum and the Golgi apparatus in *plasma cells*) or the result of a material waiting to be expelled (sebum granules in a *sebocyte*) or material that has been phagocytosed (grains of haemosiderin in the *haemosiderophage*).

The positions of the nucleus can be classified into central, paracentral or subterminal, peripheral and punched out (Figure 4).

Number of nuclei

Usually, cells have a single nucleus. However, there are special cases in which there may exist binucleate, multinucleate as well as anucleate cells (Figure 5). In mammals, an example of anucleate cell is the *erythrocyte*, in which extreme differentiation has led to the loss of the nucleus. Physiologically, multinucleation occurs when different cells of the same type merge (syncytium), however, it may also occur in conditions of inefficient cytokinesis (plasmodium). A syncytium is clearly the result of a particular cellular activity of some cytotypes (e.g. *the inflammatory giant cell*). Imperfect cytokinesis is more frequently observed in the context of pathological changes. It is a mechanism through which binucleate, rather than multinucleate, cells are typically formed. This mechanism may represent an atypical character, which will be dealt with later in this book (see Chapter 6, Morphological alterations in cells).

Chromatin patterns

Chromatin is a collection of genetic material (DNA) of cells. It also includes proteins which assist supercoiling and structural maintenance of DNA. During the resting

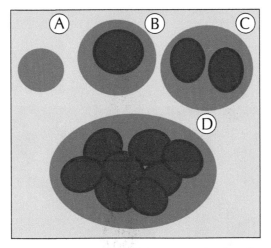

Figure 5 - Schematic representation of the number of nuclei present within the cells: non-nucleated cell (A), mononuclear cell (B), binucleated cell (C) and multinucleated cell (D).

phase, chromatin is compact and identifiable, in terms of morphology, by its intense colour (heterochromatin). During protein synthesis, DNA must be accessible to enzymes. Consequently, compact areas will no longer be visible, giving way to less stained areas, displaying finer and thinner patterns (euchromatin). An increase in chromatin characterized by sparsely stained and loose areas (euchromatin), indicates increased transcription of large areas of DNA and, therefore, cellular protein synthesis (active cell). Conversely, the presence of intensely stained compact chromatin (heterochromatin) suggests a resting state of the cell. There are special cases in which a compact chromatin pattern corresponds to extremely high protein synthesis. This is the case for the *plasma cell*, in which large aggregates of compact chromatin clash with the well-known high protein (antibodies) synthesis. The explanation of this apparent conflict lies in the fact that plasma cells, in their production and secretion of antibodies, transcribe only a small portion of their DNA, the one that encodes for the immunoglobulin of interest, leaving the rest of its genetic material supercoiled.

Under normal conditions, some cytotypes have a characteristic chromatin pattern due to their basal metabolic activity, which may be of help for their recognition. Figure 6 shows some major chromatin patterns: fine, finely stippled, lacy, coarse, clumped and compact. Overlaps between various patterns are possible. For example, it is possible to observe a finely stippled chromatin pattern together with chromatin clumps.

Nucleolus

The nucleolus hosts ribosomal RNA synthesis. Its relative hypertrophy allows it to appear generally as a round, central structure. It is chromatically different from the rest of the nuclear material, appearing bluish or sometimes of a slightly different shade of purple to that of the chromatin (Figure 7), depending on the stains. Its presence, or rather its identification within the nucleus (sometimes referred to as the *prominent nucleolus*), is a sign of cellular activity connected to protein synthesis. Some cytotypes tend to have a visible nucleolus (e.g. the *hepatocyte* and the *immunoblast*), or multiple visible nucleoli (e.g. the *centroblast*), which are specific features for their identification.

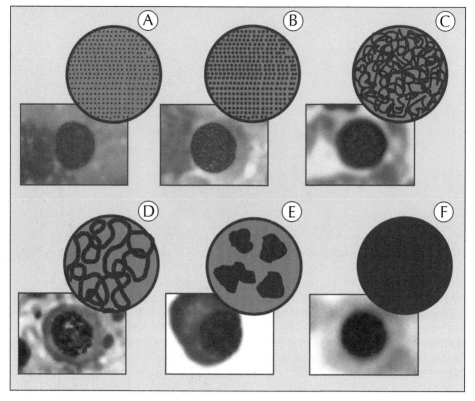

Figure 6 - Main chromatin pattern depicted using schematic representation and corresponding micropho-tographic examples: fine (A), finely stippled (B), lacy (C), coarse (D), clumped (E) and compact (F).

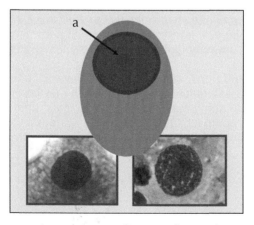

Figure 7 - Schematic representation and corresponding microphotographic examples of the position, shape and colour of the nucleolus (a).

Mitosis

Mitotic figures are specific shapes that are acquired by the nucleus when the cell undergoes cell division (Figure 8). This condition is called a *mitotic figure*. It consists of a morphological change of the nucleus, from typically round (with all the nuances

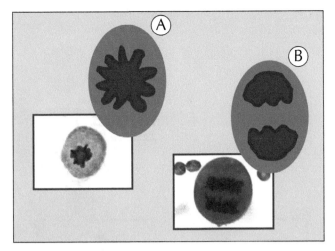

Figure 8 - Schematic representation and microphotographic corresponding examples of mitotic figures: 'explosion' mitosis (A) and mitosis with symmetrical segregation of chromatin aggregates (B).

of the shapes, see Figure 3) to star-shaped or fragmented into parts. In diagnostic cytology, a mitotic figure defines all the stages of mitosis (from prophase to telophase, as well as cytokinesis). More precisely its nucleus appears as a star-shaped or firework burst shape (Figure 8A) or as two nuclear fragments that move away from each other (Figure 8B). In cytology, a typical mitotic figure merely indicates that a cell is dividing.

The interpretation of this character is of strategic importance only if associated with the cell type it refers to. Indeed, in some cytotypes, this is to be considered absolutely normal due to a high physiological cell turnover (e.g. *immunoblast* or *basal cell*); in others, given their lower turnover, it is considered atypical (e.g. *keratinized squamous epithelial cell, chondroblast*).

■ Cytoplasmic morphologies

Cytoplasmic morphologies refer to morphological features (shape and colour) that depend on cytoplasm. They take into account:

- colour;
- pattern;
- visible intracytoplasmic structures and inclusions.

Colour of the cytoplasm

The cytoplasm can vary from greyish or, in some cases, pinkish, to an intense blue, if DiffQuik® or similar stains are being used (Figure 9). The closer the colour gets to an intense blue, the more the term 'basophilic' is used. Although this term is mistakenly used as it refers to the analogy with the colour of the haematoxylin–eosin stain, it provides, etymologically speaking, a functional meaning that justifies its sustained use. The cytoplasmic basophilia represents its affinity to stain with basic dyes. Such affinity is determined by its acidity, which, in turn, is mostly determined by the amount of ribosomal RNA present in the ribosomes of the endoplasmic

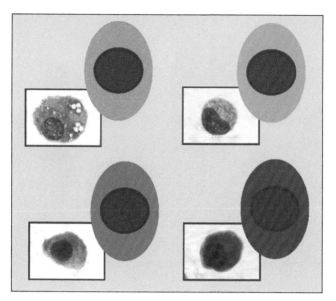

Figure 9 - Schematic representation and corresponding microphotographic examples of the different colours of the cytoplasm: eosinophilic (or pink) (A), amphophilic (or grey) (B), weakly basophilic (or blue) (C) and intensely basophilic (or deep blue) (D).

reticulum (actively involved in protein synthesis). A pink stain is mainly due to proteinaceous material, while grey suggests equally low affinity for acid or basic dyes (amphophilic). In some cases, intense staining of the cytoplasm can highlight areas that have no particular chromatic affinity; a typical example is the Golgi apparatus (e.g. *plasma cell*). The recognition of this area is used to identify some cytotypes, while the recognition of such a structure is not determined by a change of its own colour but rather by a change in the colour of the surrounding cytoplasm which highlights it. This means that, where it is visible, an evaluation of its size (relative to the total area of the cytoplasm) can also provide information about its functionality. A significant hypertrophy of the Golgi apparatus thus highlighted suggests that a considerable amount of material is being transported outside of the cell (e.g. *plasma cell* and *osteoblast*).

Pattern of the cytoplasm

Regardless of its colour, the 'pattern' of a cytoplasm refers to its shape and appearance. In general, it can vary from a 'amorphous' or 'smooth' (homogeneous), to 'granular' or 'rough'. Usually, the presence of one of these features is strongly associated with a particular cytotype (Figure 10).

Visible intracytoplasmic structures and inclusions

The cytoplasm may include visible structures (vacuoles, pigments, material from phagocytosis, etc.). These may occupy a small or a large part of the cytoplasmic area. In some cases, they may even occupy the entire cytoplasmic space available (e.g. *adipocytes*). In the latter case, the structures contained in the cytoplasm are so prominent they can even characterize the colour of the cytoplasm. In other cases (e.g. *macrophages*) the cytoplasm is not affected by this bias, therefore it is easy to chromatically characterize both the inclusions and the cytoplasm itself.

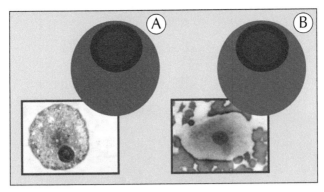

Figure 10 - Schematic examples and corresponding microphotographic representation of the different patterns of the cytoplasm: granular/rough (A) and smooth (B).

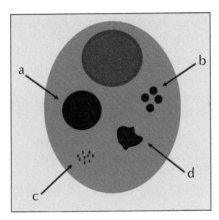

Figure 11 - Schematic representation of the morphology of intracytoplasmic inclusions: large and round, typical of vacuoles (a); small, round, typical of microvacuoles or large grains (b); fine, typical of granules (c); coarse and uneven (d).

Intracytoplasmic inclusions can have different shapes and sizes (Figure 11). Intracellular structures of cells always indicate some sort of differentiation. In the case of substances produced by a cell, such substances (e.g. proteins, hormones, pigments) may be secreted (e.g. *sebocyte*) or stored (e.g. *adipocyte*). In the case of phagocytosed substances (e.g. *macrophages*), these substances will be collected and, in some cases, digested or accumulated (e.g. *haemosiderophages*). These inclusions are extremely useful for identifying a particular cell type through the observation of its functional activity.

Some cytotypes contain specific, highly specialized, intracytoplasmic structures, which are also key for their identification (e.g. *rhabdomyocytes*, which feature contractile fibres).

■ Supercellular morphologies

The term 'supercellular morphologies' refers to those shapes that are caused by the interaction of two or more cells, in many cases resulting in the appearance of a 'cytoarchitecture' (see Chapter 4, Cytoarchitectures).

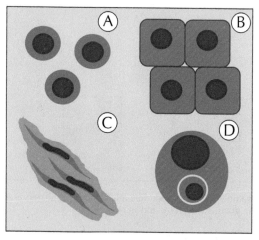

Figure 12 - Schematic representation of supercellular morphologies: no supercellular morphology (discrete cells) (A), cluster (B), aggregates (C) and phagocytic activity/emperipolesis (D).

In the context of a cytological sample, cells of the same cytotype may:

- establish no connection although they may become accumulated together in the cytological preparation due to the smearing procedure (typical of discrete cells) (Figure 12A);
- be in close and direct connection, forming aggregates, which are often referred to as *clusters* (typical of epithelial cells) (Figure 12B);
- be in close connection, which is achieved by means of matrix interposition, thus forming aggregates (typical of mesenchymal cells) (Figure 12C).

The natural tendency to establish close connections may be reduced in some cases. Such a phenomenon generally indicates an atypical feature (see Chapter 6, *Morphological alterations of cells*).

At times, cells of different cytotypes may jointly form cytoarchitetures (e.g. *ciliated epithelial cell* with *goblet cell* forming columnar cytoarchitectures in cells exfoliating from respiratory epithelium).

Some special cytotypes can establish connections with cytotypes of a different type through 'phagocytosis' in which a cell 'eats' another one (e.g. *cell-laden macrophage*) (Figure 12D), or through 'emperipolesis', which occurs when a cell engulfs another one without incorporating it into its own cytoplasm.

Distribution of cells in tissues and organs

■ Introduction

This chapter deals with the cellular elements that constitute the different organs and which, therefore, can be observed (on slides) in cytological sampling. The chapter includes figures showing the origin of the sampled cells using histological sections and diagrams, which indicate the location of the tissues/structures within the organism (Figures 13–18). The purpose of this section is to facilitate the identification of cytotypes, giving consideration to the different cytotypes that can be expected from sampling specific tissues.

Systems are composed of organs, while organs are composed of tissues, and tissues are composed of organic and inorganic acellular components, as well as cells. The components that can be sampled in a cytological investigation are, in some cases, very characteristic of the organ of origin (e.g. the *hepatocyte* from the parenchyma of the liver). Conversely, some cellular elements can be easily found in any type of organ (e.g. *fibrocytes* in the stroma of the liver or spleen or from the dermis).

Cells can be structural/resident or migrant. The cells that structurally constitute an organ will always be found in the organ itself (e.g. the *rhabdomyocyte* will always be found in skeletal muscles). On the contrary, depending on physiological/ pathological conditions, migrant cells can be found in different locations (e.g. neutrophils, which under normal conditions are found in the blood, can, if recruited by chemotactical stimulus, infiltrate inflamed tissues).

Although inflammation is a fundamental measure of the pathological condition of an organism, such status may present itself to a varying degree in normal organs, as there are cells that regularly infiltrate the tissues in small numbers to accomplish immunological surveillance. The choice to consider (in this book) as physiological those cells that are typical of an inflammatory process (a normal reactive process aimed at maintaining the body's homeostasis) stems from this concept. In most cases, so-called *inflammatory cells* are considered so not because of their morphological changes, but because they are found in different places from their normal habitat. In their normal habitat they would be considered *normal cells* (a *neutrophil* is considered normal in the blood but suggestive of inflammation if infiltrating the dermis).

Normal Cell Morphology in Canine and Feline Cytology: An Identification Guide,
First Edition. Written and translated by Lorenzo Ressel.
© 2018 John Wiley & Sons Ltd. Published 2018 by John Wiley & Sons Ltd.

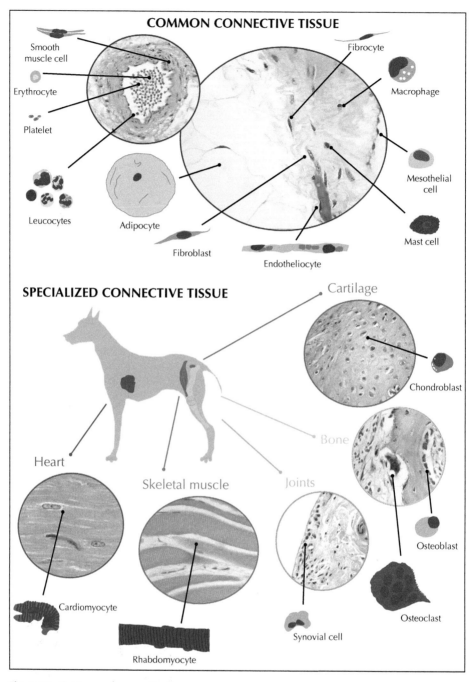

COMMON CONNECTIVE TISSUE

Smooth muscle cell

Erythrocyte

Platelet

Leucocytes

Adipocyte

Fibroblast

Endotheliocyte

Fibrocyte

Macrophage

Mesothelial cell

Mast cell

SPECIALIZED CONNECTIVE TISSUE

Cartilage

Chondroblast

Bone

Heart

Skeletal muscle

Joints

Osteoblast

Cardiomyocyte

Osteoclast

Synovial cell

Rhabdomyocyte

Figure 13 - Cytotypes of connective tissue.

Conversely, in degenerative, hyperplastic, dysplastic and neoplastic processes, cells that normally constitute tissues and organs undergo morphological alterations that produce substantial changes, or, in any case, sufficient changes to be considered pathological. This book will deal with the individual alterations which may occur during processes that include morphological cellular transformations in

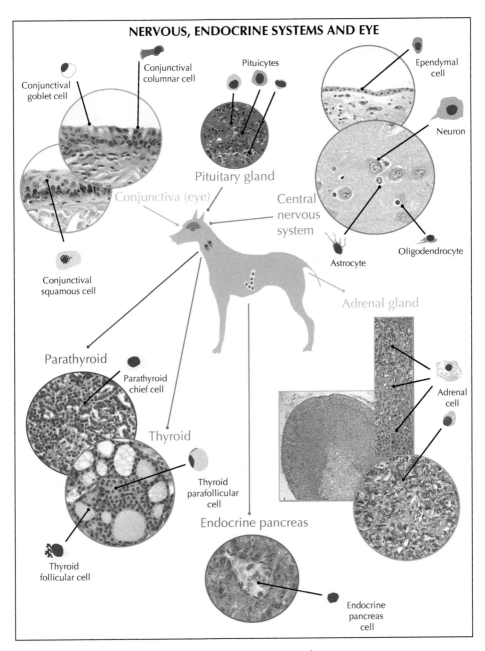

NERVOUS, ENDOCRINE SYSTEMS AND EYE

Conjunctival goblet cell

Conjunctival columnar cell

Pituicytes

Ependymal cell

Neuron

Pituitary gland

Conjunctiva (eye)

Central nervous system

Oligodendrocyte

Astrocyte

Conjunctival squamous cell

Adrenal gland

Parathyroid

Parathyroid chief cell

Adrenal cell

Thyroid

Thyroid parafollicular cell

Endocrine pancreas

Thyroid follicular cell

Endocrine pancreas cell

Figure 14 - Cytotypes of the nervous system, endocrine system and eye.

general (see Chapter 6, Morphological alterations of cells). It will not deal with the differences that may characterize cytotypes when morphologically altered. The study of pathological cytotypes, which is beyond the scope of the present discussion, is the aim of several books on diagnostic cytology, which should be consulted for additional information.

The distribution of cells in normal tissues and organs will be discussed first, and then that of inflammatory cells.

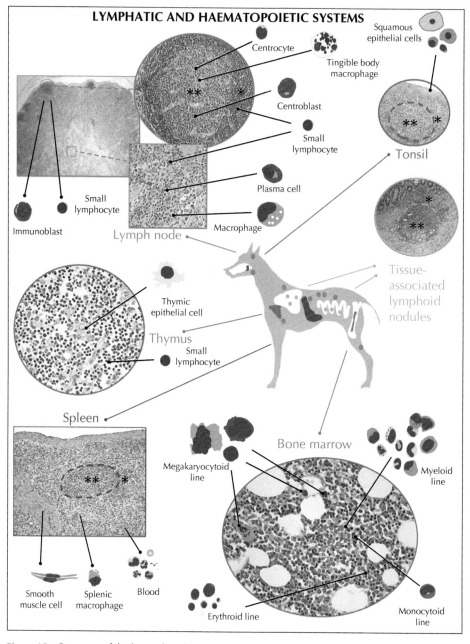

Figure 15 - Cytotypes of the haemolymphatic system *paracortex; **follicle.

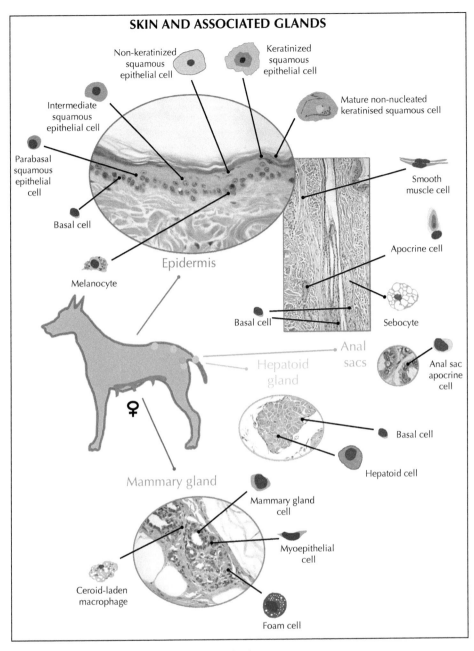

Figure 16 - Cytotypes of the skin and associated glands.

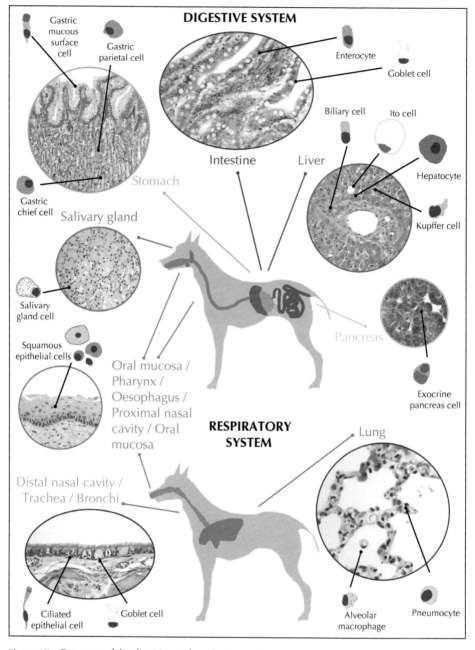

Figure 17 - Cytotypes of the digestive and respiratory systems.

■ Distribution of cells in normal tissues and organs

This section deals with the cellular components that are normally found and identified in different organs. First, the cytotypes common to all areas will be listed, and later those characteristic of each area. The aim of this section is not to provide a

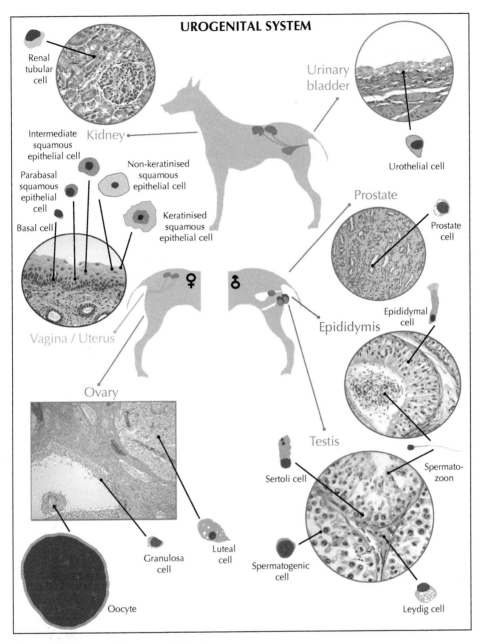

UROGENITAL SYSTEM

Renal tubular cell

Urinary bladder

Urothelial cell

Intermediate squamous epithelial cell

Kidney

Parabasal squamous epithelial cell

Non-keratinised squamous epithelial cell

Basal cell

Keratinised squamous epithelial cell

Prostate

Prostate cell

Vagina / Uterus

Epididymis

Epididymal cell

Ovary

Testis

Sertoli cell

Spermatozoon

Granulosa cell

Luteal cell

Spermatogenic cell

Oocyte

Leydig cell

Figure 18 - Cytotypes of the urogenital system.

detailed structural description of the organs from which the cells are sampled, but to provide a quick reference about the cytotypes that can be sampled. For a better insight about the structure of the individual organs, textbooks about veterinary microscopic anatomy should be consulted.

Cells that are common in tissues and organs (common connective tissue)

Some cell types are ubiquitous both in organs and systems, where they constitute the connective tissue which provides their mechanical and trophic support (or stroma).

- The connective tissue that constitutes the stroma of various organs, as well as the dermis, consists of cellular components such as *fibrocytes, fibroblasts*, as well as a small number of resident *mast cells* and *macrophages*.
- In the splanchnic cavities, pleura (chest), peritoneum (abdomen) or tunica vaginalis (scrotum) cover the contained organs and cavity walls, and are composed of lining *mesothelial cells*.
- *Smooth muscle cells* make up the involuntary muscles of both the viscera and the vessels.
- The adipose deposits present in the subcutis, adventitial tissues and body cavities are composed of *adipocytes* and rarer *lipoblasts*.
- Capillaries, common to all vascularized organs, are made of *endotheliocytes*, which may form typical capillary cytoarchitectures.
- Larger vessels are also composed of *endotheliocytes*, however, the middle contractile layer is often composed of *smooth muscle* cells.
- Blood cells are frequently found in all organ samples. This is due to vessel breakage occurring during sampling. Blood is considered a specialized connective tissue, however, since it can be found in all organs, it is included in this section. Blood is composed of cellular and acellular components. In particular, it is composed of red blood cells (*erythrocytes*) and white blood cells, which include *neutrophils, eosinophils, basophils, monocytes* and *small lymphocytes*. Furthermore, it also features *platelets*, small non-nucleated cellular elements.

Cells that are characteristic of different organs and normal systems

Some cells are characteristic of the organs from which they are sampled. However, the observation of the cytological morphology is not sufficient to categorize all the cytotypes present within a particular organ. The main cytotypes that can be easily identified through morphological observation are mentioned here.

Specialized connective tissue (cardiovascular and musculoskeletal systems)

This includes the skeletal, cardiac and muscle tissues, thus bones, cartilage and synovial membranes. These tissues can be found in different systems, such as the cardiovascular (heart) and musculoskeletal (bones, cartilage, skeletal muscles and synovia) systems.

The cardiovascular system contains the heart, which is composed of *cardiomyocytes*. The large vessels feature a muscle layer containing *smooth muscle cells*. The capillaries that can be found throughout tissues and organs typically exfoliate *endotheliocytes*, which may form characteristic capillary structures.

Skeletal muscle tissue is composed of *rhabdomyocytes*. *Osteoblasts* and *osteoclasts* can be sampled from bones, while *chondroblasts* can be sampled from cartilaginous tissue (e.g. articular cartilage). The joint cavities are covered by *synoviocytes* from the synovial membrane.

Central nervous system

Cytologically speaking, *oligodendrocytes, astrocytes* and *neurons* can be found in the central nervous system. Moreover, *ependymal cells* can be sampled from the cavities covering the central nervous system.

Endocrine system

Thyroid follicular and *thyroid parafollicular* cells can be sampled from the thyroid. The parathyroid is composed of *parathyroid chief cells*. *Adrenal cells* can be found both in the medulla and cortex of the adrenal gland, although with some differential features between sites. The glandular portion of the pituitary gland is composed of *pituicytes*. *Endocrine pancreas cells* can be found within the pancreas and constitute the islets of Langerhans.

Eye

Conjunctival columnar cells and *conjunctival goblet cells* can be sampled from the palpebral conjunctiva. The bulbar conjunctiva is composed of *conjunctival squamous cells*. The eye globe is not included in this book.

Lymph node

Several different cells, mainly from the lymphoid line, can be sampled from lymph nodes. Although precise sampling of the individual anatomical areas (cortex and medulla) appears impossible to perform, there is a certain differential distribution of the cytotypes in the two areas. *Small lymphocytes* and the rarer *immunoblasts* can be found within the para-cortex. The non-active primary follicles are composed predominantly of *small lymphocytes*. *Small lymphocytes, centrocytes, centroblasts* and (rarely) *immunoblasts* can be sampled from the active secondary follicles. *Plasma cells* can be retrieved from the medulla, where *macrophages* and *small lymphocytes* can be also observed. Within the hyperplastic lymph node, *lymphoglandular bodies* and *tingible body macrophages* are observed.

Tissue-associated lymphoid nodules

Scattered lymphatic nodules are present in various tissues and organs, notably in the respiratory and digestive systems. The population sampled is comparable to that of the cortical lymph nodes.

Thymus

Small lymphocytes and rare *thymic epithelial cells* can be sampled from the thymus gland which regresses early in adult life.

Spleen

The red pulp of the spleen consists largely of *erythrocytes* and rare *splenic macrophages*. The white pulp contains a cellular population consisting of *small lymphocytes* or, during hyperplasia, it is comparable to that of the cortical lymph node.

Bone marrow

Bone marrow is essentially composed of cells representing the erythroid and myeloid maturation lineages. *Rubriblasts, prorubricytes, rubricytes* (in their three forms: *basophilic, polychromatic* and *normochromatic*) and *metarubricytes* are part of the erythroid lineage (in order of maturation, from the least to the most mature cell type). The *polychromatophilic erythrocyte* is the immature form of the *erythrocyte*.

Myeloblasts, promyelocytes, myelocytes, metamyelocytes and *band cells* belong to the myeloid lineage leading to the granulocytes (*neutrophils, eosinophils, basophils*). *Monoblasts*, precursors of the *monocytes*, are often difficult to differentiate from the granulocytic lineage.

Megakaryoblasts, promegakaryocytes and *megakaryocytes*, belonging to the megakaryocytic lineage, are also observed.

Due to the location of the bone marrow (inside the bone), *osteoblasts* and *osteoclasts* can also be found.

Epidermis and appendages

The epidermis is mostly made of epithelial cells, which (starting from the deepest layer) are cytologically classified as *basal cells, parabasal squamous epithelial cells, intermediate squamous epithelial cells, non-keratinized squamous epithelial cells, keratinized squamous epithelial cells* and *mature non-nucleated keratinized squamous cells (or lamellar keratin)*. The hair follicle, in its deepest part, is composed of *basal cells* which are also referred as *trichoblasts*.

The glands associated with the follicles are of two types: sebaceous glands, composed of *sebocytes* and reserve *basal cells*, and apocrine glands, composed of *apocrine cells* and rare, peripheral *myoepithelial cells*. Eccrine glands are rare and a cytological counterpart is not described. In dogs, within particular subcutaneous areas, modified sebaceous glands (hepatoid glands), consisting of *hepatoid cells* and reserve *basal cells*, can be found. *Anal sac apocrine cells* can be found inside specialized structures of carnivores called anal sacs.

Mammary gland

Mammary gland cells, which constitute the ductule–alveolar structures associated with *myoepithelial cells*, are found in the mammary gland. Lactating mammary glands feature *mammary foam cells* (as an active status of *mammary gland cells*) and often *ceroid-laden macrophages*.

Ear

The external ear canal is completely covered by *basal cells, parabasal squamous epithelial cells, intermediate squamous epithelial cells* and *keratinized squamous epithelial cells*. The middle and internal ear are not discussed in this book.

Digestive system

The buccal cavity is covered by *basal cells, parabasal squamous epithelial cells, intermediate squamous epithelial cells* and *non-keratinized squamous epithelial cells*. *Rhabdomyocytes* can be detected in the tongue. The salivary glands, consisting of *salivary gland cells*, can be found at the beginning of the digestive tract.

The oesophagus is covered with the same cells as the buccal cavity and the pharynx, so there are epithelial cells at different degrees of maturation.

Depending on the sampling location, *gastric mucous surface cell*, *gastric parietal cells* and *gastric chief cells* can be found within the stomach.

The intestine is covered with *enterocytes*, interspersed with *goblet cells*.

Scattered tissue-associated lymphoid nodules are present at various levels in the different viscera.

Liver

The liver contains *hepatocytes* (constituting its parenchyma), as well as *biliary cells* and *Kupffer cells*. At times, *Ito cells* can also be found. Cells that constitute the liver capsule (Glisson's capsule) are morphologically comparable to *mesothelial cells*.

Pancreas

Exocrine pancreas cells and *endocrine pancreas cells* (see Endocrine system) can be found in the pancreas.

Respiratory system

Stratified squamous epithelial cells at different degrees of maturation can be found at the beginning of the upper respiratory tract similarly to the digestive tract. Further down (caudal nasal cavity and larynx/trachea/bronchi), *ciliated epithelial cells* are interspersed with *goblet cells*.

In the lung *pneumocytes* and *alveolar macrophages* can be found at the level of the alveoli. Scattered tissue-associated lymphoid nodules are present at different levels in the respiratory tract.

Urinary tract

Renal tubular cells and large structures that are fully comparable to the glomeruli (*see* Chapter 4, Cytoarchitectures) can be sampled from the kidney. *Urothelial cells* can be found in the bladder.

Male reproductive system

Leydig cells, *Sertoli cells*, *spermatogenic cells* and *spermatozoa* are found in the male genitalia. *Epididymal cells* and *spermatozoa* are typical of the epididymis.

Female reproductive system

Oocytes, *granulosa cells* and *luteal cells* can be found in the ovary. The epithelium of the vagina and uterus is composed of *basal cells*, *parabasal squamous epithelial cells*, *intermediate squamous epithelial cells*, *non-keratinized squamous cells* and *keratinized squamous cells*.

Distribution of cells in tissues and organs in inflammatory processes

During the inflammatory process, resident cells of the blood extravasate and infiltrate the tissues. In addition, some resident cells (e.g. resident *macrophages* and *mast cells*) may increase in numbers. Therefore, an inflamed tissue will feature (in different proportions according to the type and age of the process) *neutrophils, eosinophils, lymphocytes, macrophages* (either from blood *monocytes* or from tissue resident *macrophages*) and *plasma cells*. Plasma cells can acquire specific morphologies, such as those of *flame cells* or *Mott cells*.

Macrophages, within an inflamed area, may acquire the morphology of *microorganism-laden macrophages* when they phagocytose aetiological agents. Alternatively, if they are carrying out clearance of dying inflammatory cells, they may appear as *cell-laden macrophages*. During clearance activity, *macrophages* may also assume specific denominations depending on the material they phagocytose: melanin (*melanophage*), erythrocytes and haemosiderin (*haemosiderophage*), fat (*adipophage*). Furthermore, in special situations (e.g. granulomatous inflammation) macrophages appear as *epithelioid macrophages* or *inflammatory giant cells*.

In chronic phases of the inflammatory process, reactive *fibroblasts* may constitute the predominant component, especially during fibrosis and granulation tissue formation.

During inflammation involving the serosa, mesothelial cells become *activated mesothelial cells*.

For more detailed information about qualitative and quantitative analysis of inflammatory cytotypes, as well as their correlations with different pathological conditions, please refer to diagnostic cytology textbooks.

Cytotypes

■ Introduction

This chapter describes the different cell types (cytotypes) identifiable by cytological examination, in the form of uniformly organized 'cytotype identification sheets'. The identification sheets are characterized by the name of the cell type (Figure 19A), and are arranged in alphabetical order according to the cytotype name. Each sheet is accompanied by a photomicrograph which depicts the cell type at high magnification stained with DiffQuik® stain (Figure 19B), and by a schematic representation (diagram) based on the microphotograph (Figure 19C), which highlights the unique characteristics of the cell type useful to its identification.

In the context of the photomicrograph there is a 7 μm scale bar (Figure 19D), which is the size of a red blood cell; this represents the typical cell used to make size comparisons during microscopic observation. An erythrocyte is also shown with a 7 μm diameter in the diagram (Figure 19E).

The central part (Figure 19F) is occupied by the text, which is divided into:

- general characteristics and biological function – biological characteristics of the cell type are briefly described in order to clarify their anatomical and physiological features in normal conditions;
- shape and size – information related to shape, size and characteristics of the cell, also information related to the nuclear:cytoplasmic ratio when considered useful;
- nucleus – morphological characteristics of the nucleus and subnuclear components (chromatin, nucleoli);
- cytoplasm – morphological characteristics of the cytoplasm and its structures;
- location – anatomical locations in which the cytotype can be found;
- cytoarchitectures – information about whether the cell type usually forms architectures with other cells of the same cytotype (see Chapter 4, Cytoarchitectures);
- associated background – the type of background typically associated with the particular cytotype, if any (see Chapter 5, Background);
- differential diagnosis – other morphologically similar cell types, which can be confused with the specific cytotype, if any.

Species differences (dog vs. cat) are clarified within each section.

Normal Cell Morphology in Canine and Feline Cytology: An Identification Guide, First Edition. Written and translated by Lorenzo Ressel.

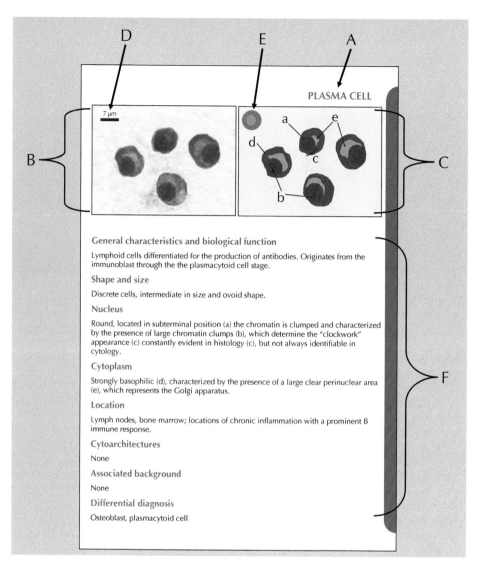

D E A

PLASMA CELL

7 μm

a e
d
c
b

B C

General characteristics and biological function

Lymphoid cells differentiated for the production of antibodies. Originates from the immunoblast through the the plasmacytoid cell stage.

Shape and size

Discrete cells, intermediate in size and ovoid shape.

Nucleus

Round, located in subterminal position (a) the chromatin is clumped and characterized by the presence of large chromatin clumps (b), which determine the "clockwork" appearance (c) constantly evident in histology (c), but not always identifiable in cytology.

Cytoplasm

Strongly basophilic (d), characterized by the presence of a large clear perinuclear area (e), which represents the Golgi apparatus.

Location

Lymph nodes, bone marrow; locations of chronic inflammation with a prominent B immune response.

Cytoarchitectures

None

Associated background

None

Differential diagnosis

Osteoblast, plasmacytoid cell

F

Figure 19 - Structure of 'cytotype identification sheets'. Name (A), microphotograph (B), schematic representation (C), scale bar (D), schematic representation of a red blood cell to scale (E), explanatory text (F).

■ Activated mesothelial cell

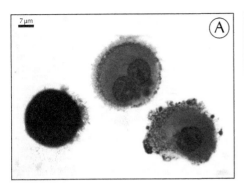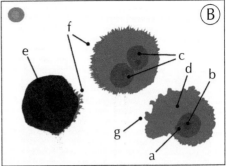

Figure 20 - Photomicrograph (A) and schematic representation (B) of the activated mesothelial cell.

General characteristics and biological function

Morphology acquired by mesothelial cell during inflammatory conditions.

Shape and size

Large cell, with a low nuclear:cytoplasmic ratio, predominantly round in shape. Physiologically exhibits a high degree of anisokaryosis and anisocytosis.

Nucleus

Round (a), with finely stippled chromatin, with evident central nucleolus (b). Often binucleated (c).

Cytoplasm

Intensely basophilic (d). In some cases, it is hyperbasophilic (e), making visualization of the nucleus difficult. Cell margins exhibit microvilli which give the characteristic appearance of an eosinophilic 'crown' radiating from the edges (f); sometimes cytoplasmic margins have characteristic blebs (g).

Location

Serosal cavities during inflammation.

Cytoarchitectures

Activated mesotheliocytes usually exfoliate individually, but, more rarely, can form small pavement clusters.

Associated background

None or proteinaceous.

Differential diagnosis

Neoplastic cells. Given the atypical features, these cells are often difficult to differentiate from those of neoplastic origin.

■ Adipocyte

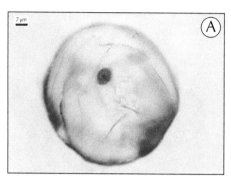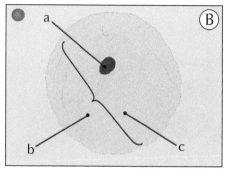

Figure 21 - Photomicrograph (A) and schematic representation (B) of the adipocyte.

General characteristics and biological function

The mature adipocyte is a mesenchymal cell which stores fat within the cytoplasm and releases it upon demand.

Shape and size

Large round cells with low nuclear:cytoplasmic ratio and characterized by a typical 'signet ring' shape.

Nucleus

Peripherally located, but it may look central or paracentral according to the position of the cell over the slide. Round to oval in shape, with compact chromatin (a).

Cytoplasm

It is almost entirely occupied by a single large unstained, optically empty lipid vacuole (b). Cracking folds (artefact) of the cytoplasmic membrane may be evident (c).

Location

The adipocyte, which represents the mature adipose tissue functional unit, can be found in any body location that is characterized by this type of connective tissue.

Cytoarchitectures

The adipocyte often forms three-dimensional solid cytoarchitectures or is found as discrete cells.

Associated background

Fat matrix.

Differential diagnosis

Shape and size are characteristic, but it can be rarely mistaken for a squamous epithelial cell or very large macrophage, in particular an adipophage.

■ Adipophage

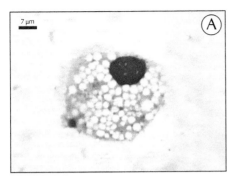
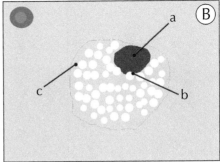

Figure 22 - Photomicrograph (A) and schematic representation (B) of the adipophage.

General features and biological function

The adipophages are macrophages phagocytosing large amounts of lipid material.

Size and shape

See Macrophage.

Nucleus

Peripherally located (a) and occasionally indented by small empty vacuoles (b).

Cytoplasm

Abundant. Characterized by large numbers of small clear vacuoles (c).

Location

The adipophages are located in areas characterized by significant clearance of lipids (adipose tissue, nervous tissue) during inflammation.

Cytoarchitectures

None.

Associated background

Fat matrix.

Differential diagnosis

Salivary gland cell, sebocyte, lipoblast.

■ Adrenal cell

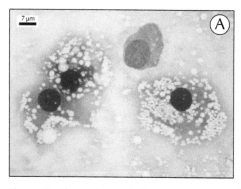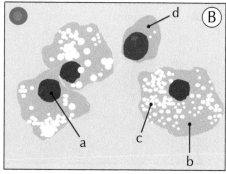

Figure 23 - Photomicrograph (A; Source: Courtesy of Carlo Masserdotti) and schematic representation (B) of the adrenal cell.

General characteristics and biological function

Endocrine cells deputed to the production of adrenal hormones. Cells derived from cortical portion (mineralocorticoids, glucocorticoids and sex hormones) and the medulla (catecholamines) are identified.

Shape and size

Large cells, with low (cortical) or intermediate (medullary) nuclear:cytoplasmic ratio, with fading cytoplasmic limits.

Nucleus

Central or subterminal and round (a), with compact to finely stippled chromatin.

Cytoplasm

Abundant (b) and rich in clear cytoplasmic vacuoles, which range from fine to medium (c) in the case of cells derived from the cortical area. More homogeneous and basophilic in medulla-derived elements (d).

Location

Adrenal gland.

Cytoarchitectures

Usually isolated, more rarely small pavement clusters.

Associated background

None.

Differential diagnosis

Macrophage.

■ Alveolar macrophage

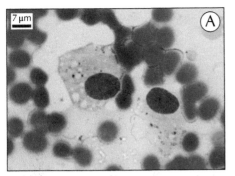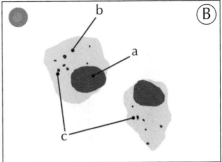

Figure 24 - Photomicrograph (A) and schematic representation (B) of the alveolar macrophage.

General characteristics and biological function

Resident macrophage of the lung, responsible for the clearance of inhaled particles.

Shape and size

See Macrophage.

Nucleus

See Macrophage (a).

Cytoplasm

See Macrophage (b). Typically, may contain small dark pigments (c), representing inhaled particles, often from dust, smoke, pollution.

Location

Lung.

Cytoarchitectures

None.

Associated background

None.

Differential diagnosis

Other macrophages containing different pigments (haemosiderophage, melanophage, ceroid-laden macrophage).

■ Anal sac apocrine cell

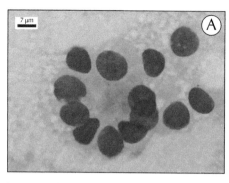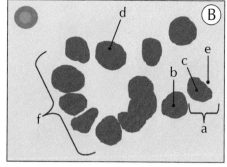

Figure 25 - Photomicrograph (A) and schematic representation (B) of the anal sac apocrine cell.

General characteristics and biological function

Epithelial cells that constitute the main elements of the modified apocrine secreting cells of the anal sacs in carnivores.

Shape and size

Small cells (a), round or polygonal, with high nuclear:cytoplasmic ratio.

Nucleus

Round (b) to ovoid (c), with fine chromatin (d).

Cytoplasm

Particularly light grey; it is often difficult to identify the cytoplasmic limits (e).

Location

Anal sacs.

Cytoarchitectures

Acinar (f), referred to as 'rosettes'.

Associated background

None.

Differential diagnosis

The apocrine cells of anal sacs retain their well-differentiated morphology in neoplastic transformation, therefore is difficult to differentiate normal from neoplastic cells of this origin.

■ Apocrine cell

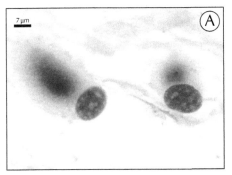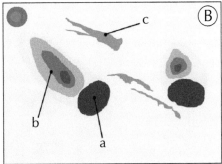

Figure 26 - Photomicrograph (A) and schematic representation (B) of the apocrine cell.

General characteristics and biological function

Epithelial apocrine secreting cell, forming apocrine glands mainly within skin but also in other areas.

Shape and size

Cells of elongated or ovoid shape, small to medium sized, with low nuclear: cytoplasmic ratio.

Nucleus

Round to ovoid and peripheral (a).

Cytoplasm

Basophilic, which can be more intense at the centre and reduced closer to the cytoplasmic limits (b).

Location

Apocrine glands.

Cytoarchitectures

They can frequently form acinar cytoarchitectures or they exfoliate as individual elements.

Associated background

Proteinaceous background (c).

Differential diagnosis

Columnar ciliated epithelial cell, osteoblast.

■ Astrocyte

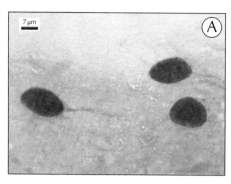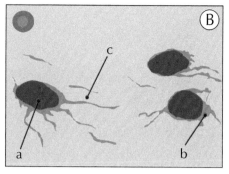

Figure 27 - Photomicrograph (A) and schematic representation (B) of the astrocyte.

General characteristics and biological function

Cells of nervous origin which provide structural and functional support to the nervous matrix and neurons.

Shape and size

Medium-sized cells, star-shaped with fine elongations. High nuclear:cytoplasmic ratio.

Nucleus

Large, vesicular, egg-shaped, with finely stippled chromatin (a).

Cytoplasm

Basophilic, scant, difficult to detect (b), extends in multiple fine cellular extensions (c), that can be barely visible due to their fragility and/or very small diameter.

Location

Central nervous system.

Cytoarchitectures

None.

Associated background

Granular proteinaceous matrix.

Differential diagnosis

Oligodendrocyte.

■ Band cell

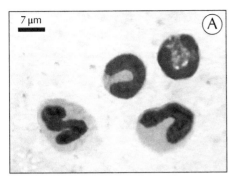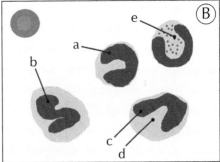

Figure 28 - Photomicrograph (A) and schematic representation (B) of the band cell.

General characteristics and biological function

Represents the maturational stage immediately before the granulocyte cytotype, whether they are neutrophils, eosinophils or basophils.

Shape and size

Small, round cell.

Nucleus

Typically not deeply lobulated, when compared with the mature form of the granulocyte, but is typically C (a), S (b) or V (c) -shaped. Chromatin is compact.

Cytoplasm

Clear, with no visible granules when a precursor of the neutrophil (d), or contains eosinophilic (e) or basophilic granules according to the myeloid maturation class (basophil or eosinophil).

Location

The band cell is normally found in the bone marrow, but it may appear in the blood in inflammation characterized by massive granulocyte recruitment.

Cytoarchitectures

None.

Associated background

None.

Differential diagnosis

Mature granulocyte, metamyelocyte, monocyte.

■ Basal cell

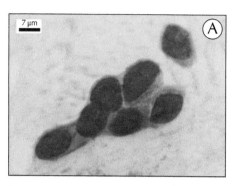 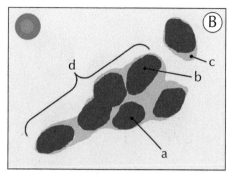

Figure 29 - Micrograph (A) and schematic representation (B) of the basal cell.

General characteristics and biological function

The term 'basal cell' indicates a group of morphologically undifferentiated epithelial cells that form the basal epithelial compartment of mucosae, epidermis, sebaceous/hepatoid glands (basaloid cells) and follicles (trichoblasts). Basal cells represent the 'stem' regenerative compartment of such structures.

Shape and size

Small cells, with a high nuclear:cytoplasmic ratio.

Nucleus

Round (a) to ovoid (b), with compact chromatin and central to paracentral location.

Cytoplasm

Scant amorphous cytoplasm, amphophilic to weakly basophilic (c) without prominent cytoplasmic structures.

Location

Basal compartment of epithelia.

Cytoarchitectures

Pavement or columnar cytoarchitectures almost always in association with the mature forms that originate from the differentiation of the basal cell. The identification of small clusters of basal cells alone (d) is suggestive of trichoblastic origin.

Associated background

None in general. Eosinophilic proteinaceous matrix is a possible finding if they originate from the hair bulb (trichoblasts).

Differential diagnosis

Due to the size and the high nuclear:cytoplasmic ratio, they may look, when not forming clusters, similar to small lymphocytes.

■ Basophil

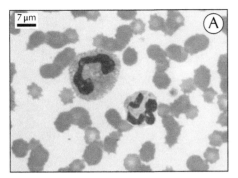
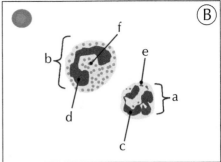

Figure 30 - Photomicrograph (A) and schematic representation (B) of the basophil.

General characteristics and biological function

Very rare circulating granulocytes, counterpart of tissue mast cells.

Shape and size

Round, 10–15 µm in the dog (a); up to 20 µm in the cat (b).

Nucleus

Lobulated, with similar morphology to the neutrophil in the dog (c); less lobulated in cats (d).

Cytoplasm

Amphophilic, characterized by scattered faint granules. Dog: the granules are not easily detectable (e). Cat: the granules are rod-shaped and greyish; similarly to eosinophil, they occupy a large portion of the cytoplasm (f).

Location

Circulating blood (very rare), haematopoietic marrow.

Cytoarchitectures

None.

Associated background

None.

Differential diagnosis

Neutrophil (dog), eosinophil (cat).

■ Basophilic rubricyte

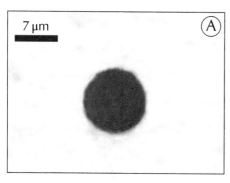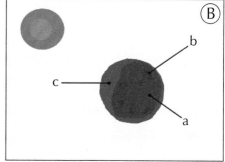

Figure 31 - Micrograph (A) and schematic representation (B) of the basophilic rubricyte.

General characteristics and biological function

Erythropoietic cell, maturing from prorubricyte to polychromatic rubricyte. It represents the first maturation stage of rubricytes.

Shape and size

Small cell, discrete, round, with a high nuclear:cytoplasmic ratio.

Nucleus

Round, central (a), with clumped chromatin (b).

Cytoplasm

Basophilic, scant (c).

Location

Bone marrow.

Cytoarchitectures

None.

Associated background

None.

Differential diagnosis

Small lymphocyte, prorubricyte, other rubricyte stages.

■ Biliary cell

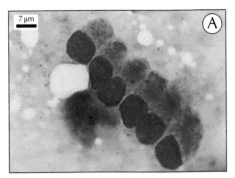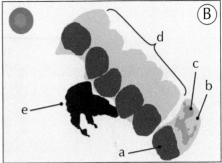

7 µm

Figure 32 - Photomicrograph (A; Source: Courtesy of Carlo Masserdotti) and schematic representation (B) of the biliary cell.

General characteristics and biological function

Cells from the epithelium of the bile ducts.

Shape and size

Small, polygonal, cuboidal to columnar cells, with intermediate nuclear:cytoplasmic ratio.

Nucleus

Peripheral, round to cuboidal, with predominantly compact chromatin (a).

Cytoplasm

Predominantly amphophilic (b), with scattered eosinophilic areas (c).

Location

Liver, bile ducts.

Cytoarchitectures

Usually, these cells exfoliate in palisades (d).

Associated background

It is possible to detect associated dark brown material, consistent with bile (e).

Differential diagnosis

In the context of the liver these cells are characteristic.

■ Cardiomyocyte

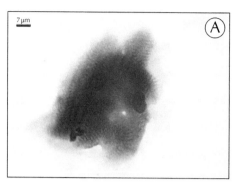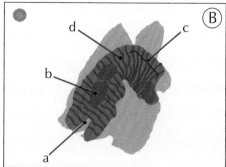

Figure 33 - Photomicrograph (A) and schematic representation (B) of the cardiomyocyte.

General characteristics and biological function

Contractile cell of the heart.

Shape and size

Elongated and branched, sometimes Y-shaped (a), diameter approximately 15 μm and length more than 85–100 μm.

Nucleus

Located in a central axial position (b), oval.

Cytoplasm

Intensely basophilic (c) and characterized by the presence of transverse bands with respect to the major axis of the cell (d).

Location

Heart.

Cytoarchitectures

These cells can exfoliate into groups forming three-dimensional cytoarchitectures.

Associated background

None.

Differential diagnosis

Rhabdomyocyte.

■ Cell-laden macrophage

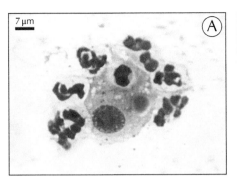 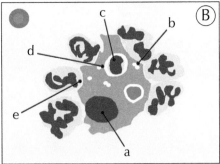

Figure 34 - Photomicrograph (A) and schematic representation (B) of the cell-laden macrophage.

General characteristics and biological function

Macrophage with phagocytic activity targeting other cells for clearance. Mainly targets aged cells or cells dying (e.g. neutrophils) as a result of pathological conditions (such as inflammation).

Shape and size

See Macrophage.

Nucleus

See Macrophage (a).

Cytoplasm

Abundant, containing optically empty vacuoles (b) and phagocytosed cells (c), often surrounded by a clear halo, which represents the phagocytic vacuole (d). Cells in the process of being phagocytosed (e) can be observed in contact with the cytoplasmic membrane.

Location

Areas rich in exuded, degenerating, inflammatory cells.

Cytoarchitectures

None.

Associated background

Proteinaceous background may be present.

Differential diagnosis

Neoplastic cells exhibiting cell cannibalism/emperipolesis.

■ Centroblast

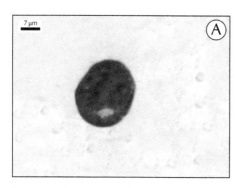
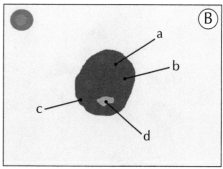

Figure 35 - Photomicrograph (A) and schematic representation (B) of the centroblast.

General characteristics and biological function

Cell of lymphoid origin, which precedes the centrocyte stage in lymphoid follicular maturation.

Shape and size

Large cell, the size of two to three erythrocytes.

Nucleus

Round and large (a), with finely stippled chromatin and characteristic presence of two to four nucleoli arranged peripherally (b).

Cytoplasm

Intensely basophilic (c), with the occasional perinuclear clear Golgi area (d).

Location

Lymph nodes and disseminated secondary lymphoid follicles.

Cytoarchitectures

None.

Associated background

None.

Differential diagnosis

Immunoblast, rubriblast.

■ Centrocyte

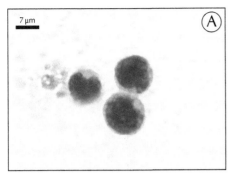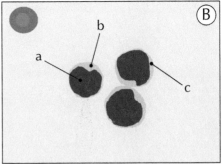

Figure 36 - Photomicrograph (A) and schematic representation (B) of the centrocyte.

General characteristics and biological function

Lymphoid cell, which follows the maturational stage of centroblast in activated lymphoid follicles.

Shape and size

Round cells with high nuclear:cytoplasmic ratio, one to two erythrocytes in size.

Nucleus

Round (a), typically with indentation (b). Chromatin less compact compared to the small lymphocyte.

Cytoplasm

Scant (but more abundant than small lymphocyte), weakly basophilic (less basophilic than the small lymphocyte) (c).

Location

Lymph node and scattered lymphoid follicles.

Cytoarchitectures

None.

Associated background

None.

Differential diagnosis

Small lymphocyte, rubricyte.

■ Ceroid-laden macrophage

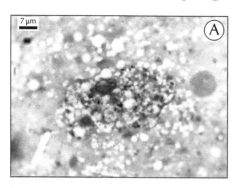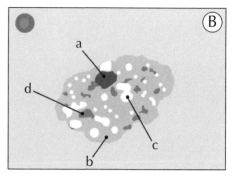

Figure 37 - Photomicrograph (A) and schematic representation (B) of the ceroid-laden macrophage.

General characteristics and biological function

Macrophage responsible for the phagocytosis of material derived from active glands (in particular, the mammary gland) or other tissues.

Shape and size

See Macrophage.

Nucleus

See Macrophage (a).

Cytoplasm

See Macrophage (b). Characterized by the simultaneous presence of optically empty vacuoles (c) and ceroid pigments of brown–green colour, angled and irregular, with variable size and shape (d).

Location

Mammary gland in secretory activity.

Cytoarchitectures

None.

Associated background

Fat–proteinaceous background.

Differential diagnosis

Other macrophages containing different pigments (haemosiderophage, melanophage).

■ Chondroblast

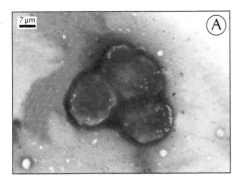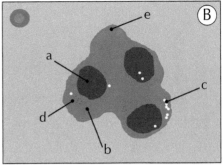

Figure 38 - Photomicrograph (A) and schematic representation (B) of the chondroblast.

General characteristics and biological function

Resident mesenchymal cell of cartilage, producing chondroid matrix.

Shape and size

Large cell, from round to oval to pear-shaped, appearing as a discrete cell with low nuclear:cytoplasmic ratio.

Nucleus

Round or ovoid, characterized by compact or finely stippled chromatin, and no prominent nucleoli (a).

Cytoplasm

Abundant, basophilic (b), characterized by the presence of scattered small to medium-sized clear vacuoles (c) and eosinophilic fine granulations (d).

Location

Cartilage.

Cytoarchitectures

None.

Associated background

Chondroid matrix (e).

Differential diagnosis

Osteoblast.

■ Ciliated epithelial cell

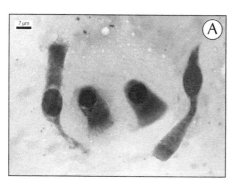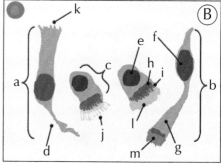

Figure 39 - Photomicrograph (A; Source: Courtesy of Carlo Masserdotti) and schematic representation (B) of the ciliated epithelial cell.

General characteristics and biological function

Lining cells of mucous membranes, such as the respiratory mucosa.

Shape and size

Elongated, columnar (a) sometimes 'wavy'. The nucleus may protrude over the cell contour (b). Sometimes they may also be more cuboidal (c). Often, there is a 'cone-shaped' basally located cell area (d) interpreted by some cytologists as an artefact.

Nucleus

From round (e) to oval (f), localized in the terminal to subterminal position, with compact to finely stippled chromatin.

Cytoplasm

Moderately basophilic (g), characterized by apical structures (ciliary apparatus) including the basal apparatus, evident as a focal hyperbasophilic area (h), with a more superficial eosinophilic zone (i) and the cilia (j). This complex structure may not be evident due to cell damage during preparation (k), or may appear more indistinct and similar to a band (l). Pink proteinaceous material can be detected in association with the cilia (m).

Location

Respiratory mucosa, conjunctiva.

Cytoarchitectures

Exfoliate as individual cells or may form small palisade cytoarchitectures in combination with basal cells and goblet cells.

Associated background

Mucinous matrix, especially from the respiratory mucosa.

Differential diagnosis

None.

■ Conjunctival columnar cell

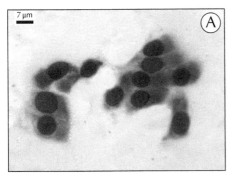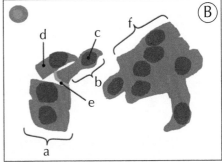

Figure 40 - Photomicrograph (A) and schematic representation (B) of the conjunctival columnar cell.

General characteristics and biological function

Epithelial cells lining the palpebral conjunctiva.

Shape and size

These are basically ciliated epithelial cells of the conjunctiva, which present both in cuboidal (a) or more columnar (b) forms.

Nucleus

Peripheral or subterminal (c), ovoid and characterized by compact chromatin.

Cytoplasm

Moderately basophilic to basophilic (d), smooth. The cilia are not always clearly detectable in cytological preparations (e).

Location

Palpebral conjunctiva.

Cytoarchitectures

These exfoliate alone or in small palisade clusters (f), together with conjunctival goblet cells.

Associated background

None.

Differential diagnosis

In general indistinguishable from other ciliated epithelial cells, sometimes more cuboidal and less elongated.

■ Conjunctival goblet cell

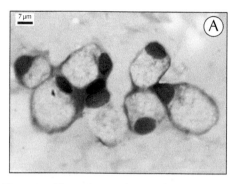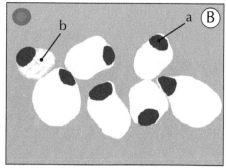

Figure 41 - Photomicrograph (A) and schematic representation (B) of the conjunctival goblet cell.

General characteristics and biological function

Goblet cells of the conjunctiva of the eyelid.

Shape and size

Cells of intermediate size, typical 'goblet' morphology, low nuclear:cytoplasmic ratio.

Nucleus

Located in a peripheral position (a), ranging from round to flat/ovoid in shape, characterized by compact chromatin.

Cytoplasm

Abundant, clear, packed with usually clear secretory granules (b).

Location

Palpebral conjunctiva.

Cytoarchitectures

These exfoliate cells alone or in small clusters along with conjunctival columnar cells.

Associated background

None.

Differential diagnosis

Indistinguishable from other goblet cells from other areas.

■ Conjunctival squamous cell

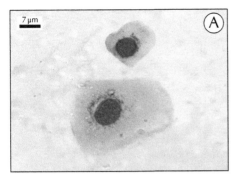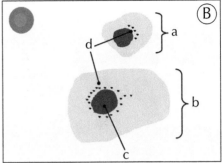

Figure 42 - Photomicrograph (A) and schematic representation (B) of the conjunctival squamous cell.

General characteristics and biological function

Epithelial cells lining part of the bulbar conjunctiva.

Shape and size

There are two main categories: intermediate, smaller cells (a), and superficial, larger cells (b). The morphology of these cells is polygonal, with a low nuclear:cytoplasmic ratio.

Nucleus

Central, characterized by compact fine chromatin (c).

Cytoplasm

Clear, amphophilic, may contain melanin pigments in the perinuclear area (d).

Location

Bulbar conjunctiva.

Cytoarchitectures

As single cells or organized in small pavement clusters.

Associated background

None.

Differential diagnosis

None.

■ Endocrine pancreas cell

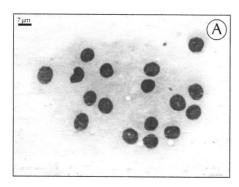 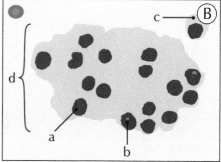

Figure 43 - Micrograph (A) and schematic representation (B) of the endocrine pancreas cell.

General characteristics and biological function

Endocrine cell of the islets of Langerhans within the pancreas. Responsible for the production of insulin, glucagon and other substances such as somatostatin and pancreatic peptide.

Shape and size

Medium-sized, round in shape.

Nucleus

Round, with compact chromatin (a) and small nucleolus occasionally visible (b).

Cytoplasm

Finely granular (c) with poorly defined cell margins, often indistinguishable from the background, leading to the 'naked nucleus' appearance.

Location

Pancreatic islets of Langerhans.

Cytoarchitectures

Can exfoliate as discrete cells but also in small pavement clusters (d).

Associated background

None.

Differential diagnosis

Other endocrine cells (thyroid follicular cell, parathyroid chief cell).

■ Endotheliocyte

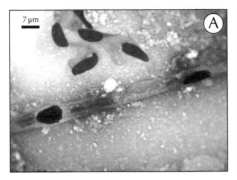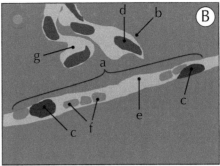

Figure 44 - Photomicrograph (A) and schematic representation (B) of the endotheliocyte.

General characteristics and biological function

Cells that form the inner lining of blood vessels.

Shape and size

Elongated and flattened cells, connected to each other and observable in the context of capillary structures formed by the folding of their membrane (a), or more rarely as individual elements, which are clearly flattened, thin or fusiform (b).

Nucleus

Flattened and fusiform and placed at the periphery of the capillary channel formed (c). It appears central in individual elements (d).

Cytoplasm

Clear, forms a canalicular structure (e) within which erythrocytes are often detected (f). In single elements cytoplasm is clear and abundant (g).

Location

Most of the tissues, in particular richly vascularized ones.

Cytoarchitectures

They form typical capillaries, which represent the core of the perivascular cytoarchitecture.

Associated background

Blood.

Differential diagnosis

Very characteristic when forming capillary structures. When detected as a single cell can appear similar to the mesothelial cell, due to its flat shape. When predominantly spindloid, it can be indistinguishable from other spindle cells (fibrocyte, fibroblast).

■ Enterocyte

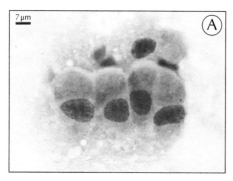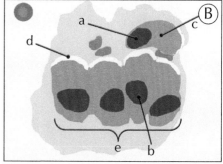

Figure 45 - Photomicrograph (A) and schematic representation (B) of the enterocyte.

General characteristics and biological function

Intestinal epithelial cell whose function is absorption of nutrients.

Shape and size

Columnar morphology, with apical microvilli.

Nucleus

Ovoid (a) or round (b), basally located in subterminal position.

Cytoplasm

Abundant, moderately basophilic (c), with apical microvilli, evident as a clear to mildly eosinophilic band (d).

Location

Digestive tract, intestinal mucosa.

Cytoarchitectures

Enterocytes exfoliate in palisade (e) or honeycomb cytoarchitectures.

Associated background

Proteinaceous.

Differential diagnosis

None.

■ Eosinophil

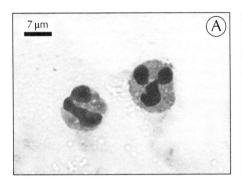
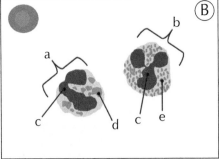

Figure 46 - Photomicrograph (A) and schematic representation (B) of the eosinophil.

General characteristics and biological function

Circulating cell, involved in allergic reactions, parasitic conditions and chronic inflammation.

Shape and size

Round, discrete cell, 10–15 µm in diameter in both the dog (a) and the cat (b).

Nucleus

Usually segmented into two lobes in the dog, or in more (but smaller number than neutrophil) in the cat (c). Chromatin is condensed to clumped.

Cytoplasm

Amphophilic. Dog: the granules vary in size, and they have a typical orange colour and do not fill the cytoplasm (d). Cat: granules are rod-shaped, more grey–orange (e).

Location

Circulating blood, bone marrow, inflammatory processes within the tissues.

Cytoarchitectures

None.

Associated background

None.

Differential diagnosis

Neutrophil, basophil.

CYTOTYPES

■ Ependymal cell

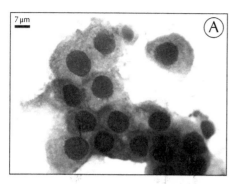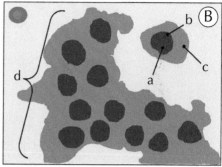

Figure 47 - Photomicrograph (A) and schematic representation (B) of the ependymal cell.

General characteristics and biological function

The ependymal cells form the epithelial-like lining of the cavity of the central nervous system.

Shape and size

Medium-sized cell, with a round shape, low nuclear:cytoplasmic ratio.

Nucleus

Round, characterized by finely granular to lacy chromatin (a), with a small nucleolus (b).

Cytoplasm

Basophilic, granular and rather abundant (c), with no particular detectable structure. The cilia, which are observed in histological specimens, are only rarely identified in cytological samples.

Location

Central nervous system.

Cytoarchitectures

Pavement to honeycomb cytoarchitectures (d).

Associated background

None.

Differential diagnosis

In the context of the central nervous system, these cells are unique in their ability of forming clusters.

■ Epididymal cell

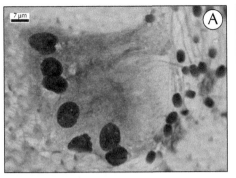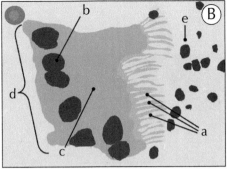

Figure 48 - Photomicrograph (A) and schematic representation (B) of the epididymal cell.

General characteristics and biological function

Cells responsible for the maturation of spermatozoa in the epididymis.

Shape and size

Columnar cells, with low nuclear:cytoplasmic ratio, characterized by apical stereocilia (a).

Nucleus

Round, with coarse to compact chromatin, located basally to subterminally (b).

Cytoplasm

Abundant, moderately basophilic (c).

Location

Male genitalia, epididymis.

Cytoarchitectures

Epididymal cells usually exfoliate in palisade cytoarchitectures (d), and are often associated with spermatozoa (e).

Associated background

Often associated with spermatozoa nuclei in the background (e).

Differential diagnosis

They can be confused with Sertoli cells. The distinctive characters, in this case, are the presence of stereocilia and hyperchromatic nucleus.

■ Epithelioid macrophage

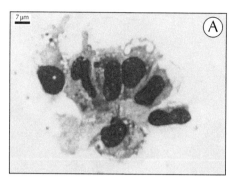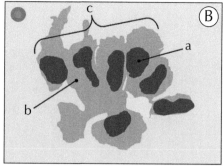

Figure 49 - Photomicrograph (A) and schematic representation (B) of the epithelioid macrophage.

General characteristics and biological function

Macrophage with an epithelial-like morphology, forming palisade clusters during granulomatous inflammation.

Shape and size

See Macrophage.

Nucleus

See Macrophage (a).

Cytoplasm

See Macrophage (b).

Location

Associated with areas affected by granulomatous-type inflammation.

Cytoarchitectures

Forms palisade, or more rarely pavement, cytoarchitectures (c).

Associated background

None or possibly proteinaceous if necrotic material is present.

Differential diagnosis

Clusters of epithelial cells. The typical macrophage morphology of associated isolated cells, the pleomorphic shape with foamy cytoplasm, and the context in which these are observed (granulomatous inflammation), help classification.

Erythrocyte

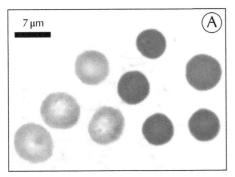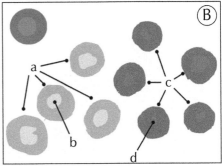

Figure 50 - Photomicrograph (A) and schematic representation (B) of the erythrocyte.

General characteristics and biological function

Terminally differentiated haematopoietic cells, derived from polychromatophilic erythrocyte. Erythrocytes (red blood cells) carry oxygen to tissues and organs through the circulatory system.

Shape and size

Small, round, non-nucleated. Dog (a): 7 µm in diameter, evident central concavity (b). Cat (c): diameter 6 µm, central concavity less evident (d).

Nucleus

Absent.

Cytoplasm

With no visible structures, characterized by a concavity in the centre (where the nucleus would be). The colour of the cytoplasm, traditionally orange, may look greenish or brownish due to staining after suboptimal fixation conditions.

Location

Circulating blood, blood collections (e.g. haematoma). They are ubiquitous in cytological preparations, in particular where blood contamination is an artefact.

Cytoarchitectures

None.

Associated background

None.

Differential diagnosis

Polychromatophilic erythrocyte.

■ Exocrine pancreas cell

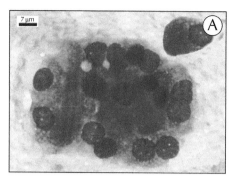
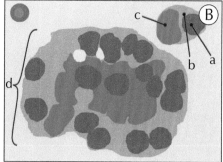

Figure 51 - Micrograph (A; Source: Courtesy of Carlo Masserdotti) and schematic representation (B) of the exocrine pancreas cell.

General characteristics and biological function

Secreting cell of the pancreas, producing pancreatic enzymes.

Shape and size

Triangular or pear-shaped, medium in size.

Nucleus

Round, located at the base of the cell (peripheral), compact to finely stippled chromatin (a).

Cytoplasm

Moderately basophilic closer to the nucleus (b), darker and more eosinophilic closer to the apical portion of the cell (c), due to the presence of zymogen granules.

Location

Pancreas.

Cytoarchitectures

Acinar cytoarchitectures (d).

Associated background

None.

Differential diagnosis

None.

■ Fibroblast

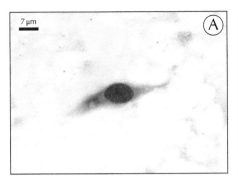 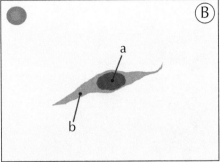

Figure 52 - Photomicrograph (A) and schematic representation (B) of the fibroblast.

General characteristics and biological function

Activated mesenchymal cell, responsible for the production of collagen and involved in granulation tissue formation.

Shape and size

Spindle cells, intermediate in size.

Nucleus

Fine to finely stippled chromatin, typically elongated/egg-shaped (a) (rounder than that of fibrocyte).

Cytoplasm

Bipolar, scant (but more abundant than in fibrocyte), basophilic (b).

Location

Connective tissue, areas of reactivity (e.g. granulation tissue) or collagen production.

Cytoarchitectures

Fibroblasts can form cellular storiform cytoarchitectures together with the matrix produced.

Associated background

Collagenous matrix.

Differential diagnosis

Fibrocyte, smooth muscle cell, myoepithelial cell.

■ Fibrocyte

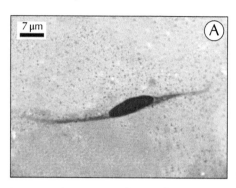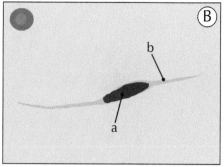

Figure 53 - Photomicrograph (A) and schematic representation (B) of the fibrocyte.

General characteristics and biological function

The most common cell in mature connective tissue, represents a quiescent fibroblast (not prominently involved in collagen formation).

Shape and size

Very thin, elongated spindle cell.

Nucleus

Heterochromatic, with condensed chromatin, central, fusiform (a).

Cytoplasm

Very scant, bipolar, moderately basophilic (b).

Location

Mature connective tissue.

Cytoarchitectures

Can form storiform cytoarchitectures together with collagen matrix.

Associated background

Collagenous matrix.

Differential diagnosis

Fibroblast, smooth muscle cell, endotheliocyte.

■ Flame cell

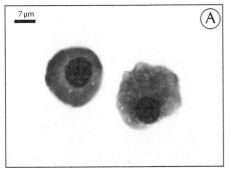
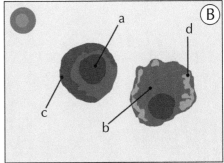

Figure 54 - Photomicrograph (A) and schematic representation (B) of the flame cell.

General characteristics and biological function

Particular type of plasma cell, which may be found in reactive conditions and in some plasmacytic proliferative disorders.

Shape and size

Oval to round in shape, or slightly pleomorphic. Larger than the plasma cell. The nuclear:cytoplasmic ratio is low.

Nucleus

Round, ranging from peripheral to subterminal (a). The chromatin pattern is typically clumped, as in plasma cells.

Cytoplasm

Basophilic, tending towards deep purple (b) compared to the plasma cell. It is characterized by purple (c) to pink (d) areas localized at the periphery of the cytoplasm.

Location

Bone marrow, areas of inflammation characterized by strong production of immunoglobulins.

Cytoarchitectures

None.

Associated background

None.

Differential diagnosis

Macrophage, plasma cell.

■ Gastric chief cell

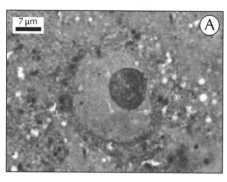 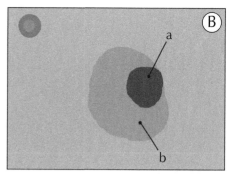

Figure 55 - Photomicrograph (A) and schematic representation (B) of the gastric chief cell.

General characteristics and biological function

Gastric cell producing pepsin.

Shape and size

Round to ovoid, with low nuclear:cytoplasmic ratio.

Nucleus

Round, paracentral to peripheral (a), with lacy to finely granular chromatin.

Cytoplasm

Basophilic, granular and abundant (b).

Location

Stomach, fundic region.

Cytoarchitectures

None.

Associated background

Proteinaceous granular background.

Differential diagnosis

Gastric parietal cell, macrophage.

■ Gastric mucous surface cell

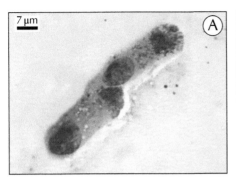
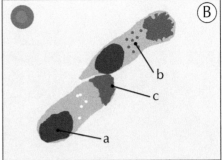

7 µm

Ⓐ

Ⓑ

b

c

a

Figure 56 - Photomicrograph (A) and schematic representation (B) of the gastric mucous surface cell.

General characteristics and biological function

Superficial lining cell of the gastric mucosa.

Shape and size

Columnar, medium-sized, with a low nuclear:cytoplasmic ratio.

Nucleus

Located at the base of the cell (peripheral), from round to oval (a), with lacy to finely granular chromatin.

Cytoplasm

Moderately basophilic, containing mucinous secretions (b), which are particularly evident at the apex of the cell (c).

Location

Stomach.

Associated background

Proteinaceous granular background.

Cytoarchitectures

Often arranged in honeycomb cytoarchitectures.

■ Gastric parietal cell

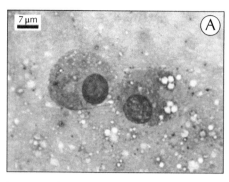 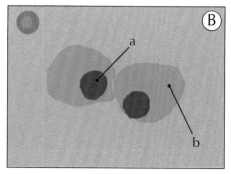

Figure 57 - Photomicrograph (A) and schematic representation (B) of the gastric parietal cell.

General characteristics and biological function

Gastric mucosal cell producing hydrochloric acid.

Shape and size

Larger than other gastric cells, with low nuclear:cytoplasmic ratio.

Nucleus

Round, paracentral to terminal (a), with clumped to lacy chromatin.

Cytoplasm

Eosinophilic (b) and granular.

Location

The stomach, especially fundic region.

Cytoarchitectures

None.

Associated background

Proteinaceous granular background.

Differential diagnosis

Gastric chief cell, macrophage.

■ Goblet cell

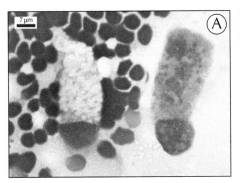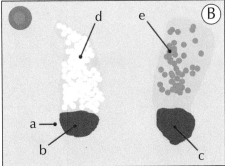

Figure 58 - Photomicrograph (A) and schematic representation (B) of the goblet cell.

General characteristics and biological function

Unicellular glands producing substances rich in mucin in mucosal surfaces.

Shape and size

Cells of intermediate to large size, with typical 'goblet' morphology and low nuclear:cytoplasmic ratio.

Nucleus

Peripheral (a), with a shape that varies from ovoid–flattened (b) to round (c), depending on the pressure exerted by the secretion produced.

Cytoplasm

Abundant, full of small granules that may appear optically empty (d) or purple (e).

Location

Mucosal surfaces.

Cytoarchitectures

These cells can exfoliate in the context of palisade cytoarchitectures together with ciliated epithelial cells.

Associated background

None.

Differential diagnosis

Adipophage, mammary foam cell, columnar epithelial cell.

■ Granular lymphocyte

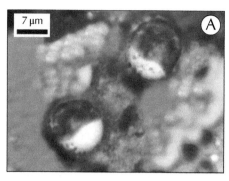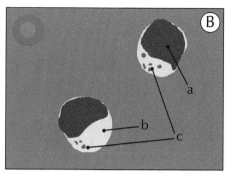

Figure 59 - Photomicrograph (A) and schematic representation (B) of the granular lymphocyte.

General characteristics and biological function

Rare lymphoid cell believed to belong to the category of killer (K) and natural killer (NK) or T cytotoxic.

Shape and size

Round cell, discrete, medium–large, with high nuclear:cytoplasmic ratio, lower than that of small lymphocyte.

Nucleus

Large, round or slightly kidney-shaped, with clumped chromatin, occupies about half of the cell (a).

Cytoplasm

Clear (b) containing variably sized, abundant to rare, pink granules (c).

Location

Very rare in normal conditions. Found in many tissues including mucous membranes.

Cytoarchitectures

None.

Associated background

None.

Differential diagnosis

Small lymphocytes, centrocyte.

■ Granulosa cell

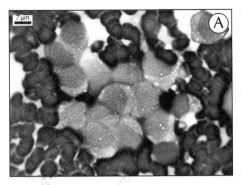 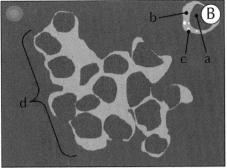

Figure 60 - Photomicrograph (A) and schematic representation (B) of the granulosa cell.

General characteristics and biological function

Cell involved in oocyte maturation and support.

Shape and size

Cuboidal cells, small, with high–intermediate nuclear:cytoplasmic ratio.

Nucleus

Polygonal, with reticular chromatin, peripheral, in contact with the cell edge (a).

Cytoplasm

Scant and basophilic (b), sometimes containing small, optically empty vacuoles (c).

Location

Female genital tract, ovary.

Cytoarchitectures

Follicular granulosa cells may form small pavement clusters (d).

Associated background

None.

Differential diagnosis

Immature lymphoid cells.

■ Haemosiderophage

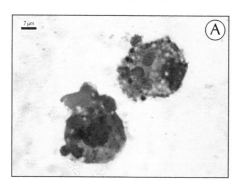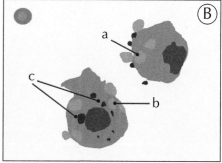

Figure 61 - Photomicrograph (A) and schematic representation (B) of the haemosiderophage.

General characteristics and biological function

Macrophage characterized by phagocytosis of erythrocytes and subsequent haemosiderin pigment accumulation. If only red blood cells are identified the name 'haemophagocyte' is used.

Shape and size

See Macrophage.

Nucleus

See Macrophage.

Cytoplasm

Characterized by still recognizable erythrocytes (a) or parts of them (b) and the dark blue pigment granules characteristic of haemosiderin (c).

Location

Reticuloendothelial system, drainage areas of blood collections (e.g. haematomas).

Cytoarchitectures

None.

Associated background

Blood.

Differential diagnosis

Melanophage, macrophage, ceroid-laden macrophage.

◼ Hepatocyte

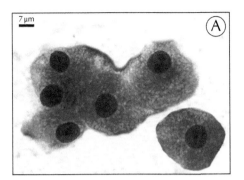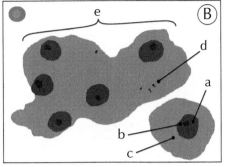

Figure 62 - Photomicrograph (A) and schematic representation (B) of the hepatocyte.

General characteristics and biological function

Epithelial cell forming the main element of the liver parenchyma. Involved in exocrine secretion, detoxification and synthesis of plasma proteins.

Shape and size

Polygonal cell, large, with a low nuclear:cytoplasmic ratio.

Nucleus

Round, central to paracentral, with compact or finely reticular chromatin (a), characterized typically by a single nucleolus (b). Occasionally, binucleated hepatocytes are detectable.

Cytoplasm

Eosinophilic, granular (c). In normal conditions rare dark granules of bile pigment and/or lipofuscin (d) can be identified.

Location

Liver.

Cytoarchitectures

Hepatocytes exfoliate usually in small clusters with pavement (e) or larger clusters with trabecular morphology.

Associated background

None.

Differential diagnosis

Highly characteristic cell. Similar to hepatoid cell, but the latter exfoliate from different locations.

■ Hepatoid cell

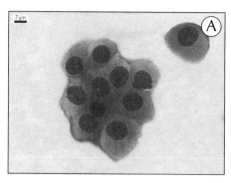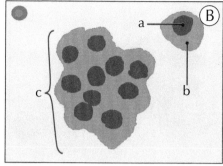

Figure 63 - Photomicrograph (A) and schematic representation (B) of the hepatoid cell.

General characteristics and biological function

Modified sebaceous gland cells of the dog. Commonly referred as 'hepatoid' (or 'peri-anal'), they owe their name to the similarity they have with the hepatocytes (it might seem more correct to use the term 'hepatocytoid').

Shape and size

Large oval or polygonal, with a low nuclear:cytoplasmic ratio.

Nucleus

Round, predominantly central, characterized by finely granular chromatin (a).

Cytoplasm

Basophilic, finely granular, similar to that of hepatocytes (b).

Location

Subcutaneous within perianal, back and tail areas.

Cytoarchitectures

Often form pavement cytoarchitectures (c), in association with basal cells, which constitute hepatoid reserve cells.

Associated background

None.

Differential diagnosis

From their morphology, these cells can be misinterpreted as hepatocytes, but the location makes confusion between the two cell types impossible.

■ Immunoblast

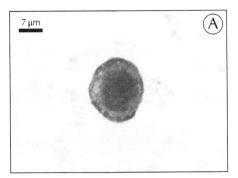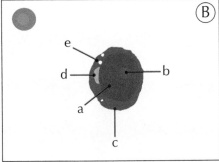

Figure 64 - Photomicrograph (A) and schematic representation (B) of the immunoblast.

General characteristics and biological function

Activated lymphoid cell that will subsequently mature into memory B cell or plasma cell through the plasmacytoid cell stage (B cell lineage), or into activated/memory T lymphocyte (T cell lineage).

Shape and size

Very large cell, discrete, typically 'rugby-ball' shaped.

Nucleus

Round, large, central (a), with finely stippled, or occasionally focally coarse chromatin with a characteristic single large central nucleolus (b). Mitotic figures are common.

Cytoplasm

Scant but rather abundant for a lymphoid cell, basophilic (c). A perinuclear Golgi area (d) is often evident, and occasionally some small vacuoles (e) are detectable. Immunoblasts of T cell lineage may have more amphophilic (grey) cytoplasm compared those of B cell lineage.

Location

Lymph node and tissue-associated lymphatic nodules: mainly in the paracortical area.

Cytoarchitectures

None.

Associated background

None.

Differential diagnosis

Centroblast, rubriblast.

■ Inflammatory giant cell

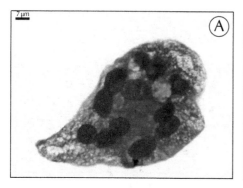 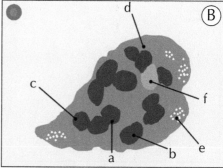

Figure 65 - Photomicrograph (A) and schematic representation (B) of the inflammatory giant cell.

General characteristics and biological function

Inflammatory giant cells are derived from the fusion of macrophages (syncitia) involved in granuloma formation.

Shape and size

Very large cells of pleomorphic shape.

Nucleus

These cells exhibit multiple nuclei, from round (a) to oval (b), arranged randomly within the cytoplasm. These nuclei are usually quite similar to each other and exhibit no anisokaryosis. The chromatin of the nuclei is finely stippled, with occasional chromatin clumps, and nucleoli are sometimes visible (c).

Cytoplasm

Basophilic (d) and sometimes occupied by small, optically empty vacuoles (e). It is sometimes possible to observe clear large areas within the cytoplasm due to fusion of phagocytic vacuoles (f), which can also occupy the centre of the cell.

Location

Commonly found in areas with granulomatous inflammation (e.g. foreign-body reactions) in association with macrophages, lymphocytes, plasma cells and granulocytes.

Cytoarchitectures

None.

Associated background

None.

Differential diagnosis

Osteoclast, megakaryocyte.

Intermediate squamous epithelial cell

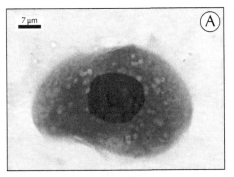 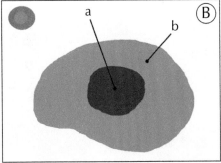

Figure 66 - Photomicrograph (A) and schematic representation (B) of the intermediate squamous epithelial cell.

General characteristics and biological function

Epithelial lining cell of stratified epithelia that represents the maturational stage subsequent to the parabasal squamous epithelial cell and antecedent to the non-keratinized squamous epithelial cell.

Shape and size

Large round cell, with no clear angular edges, and characterized by low nuclear: cytoplasmic ratio.

Nucleus

Central, rather large, round, characterized by predominantly compact chromatin pattern (a).

Cytoplasm

Abundant (b) and eosinophilic.

Location

Epithelia. In particular, this cell type from vaginal epithelium is important in assessment of cycle phases.

Cytoarchitectures

Found as individual cells or forms pavement cytoarchitectures.

Associated background

None.

Differential diagnosis

Non-keratinized squamous epithelial cell.

■ Ito cell

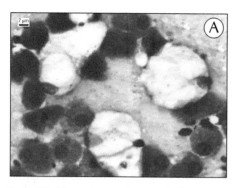 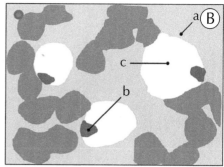

Figure 67 - Photomicrograph (A) and schematic representation (B) of the Ito cell.

General characteristics and biological function

Quiescent liver cell that becomes visible due to the accumulation of lipid containing vitamin A.

Shape and size

Unrecognizable when quiescent, they are round in shape and large in size (a) when active.

Nucleus

Oval/round, peripheral, with compact chromatin (b).

Cytoplasm

Abundant and optically empty (c).

Location

Liver

Cytoarchitectures

Usually form pavement clusters together with hepatocytes.

Associated background

None.

Differential diagnosis

Adipocyte, degenerated hepatocyte.

■ Keratinized squamous epithelial cell

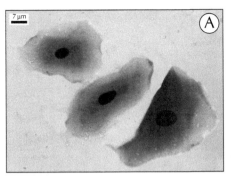 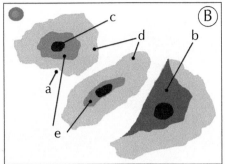

Figure 68 - Photomicrograph (A) and schematic representation (B) of the keratinized squamous epithelial cell.

General characteristics and biological function

Epithelial lining cell of stratified epithelia (e.g. epidermis). Cytoplasm is almost completely filled by keratin. It follows the stage of the non-keratinized squamous epithelial cell and precedes the stage of mature non-nucleated keratinized squamous cell.

Shape and size

Very large cell, clearly polygonal in shape, with clear detectable angular edges (a). These cells are very flattened and sometimes they may appear folded back on themselves (b).

Nucleus

Central, from round to oval, and constantly compact to pyknotic (c).

Cytoplasm

Clearer at the cell periphery (d) and darker getting closer to the perinuclear zone (e), due to the different thickness of the cell in the two zones.

Location

Superficial layers of keratinized epithelia.

Cytoarchitectures

Exfoliates as single cells or grouped in small pavement clusters.

Associated background

None.

Differential diagnosis

None.

■ Kupffer cell

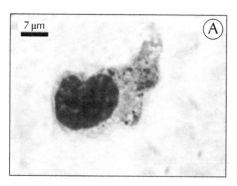
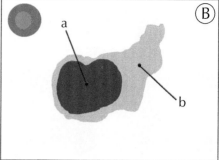

Figure 69 - Photomicrograph (A) and schematic representation (B) of the Kupffer cell.

General characteristics and biological function

Resident macrophage in the liver.

Shape and size

Medium-sized cell, with pleomorphic morphology, low nuclear:cytoplasmic ratio.

Nucleus

Kidney-shaped or ovoid, similar to that of macrophages (a).

Cytoplasm

Abundant, granular/rough, weakly basophilic to amphophilic (b).

Location

Liver.

Cytoarchitectures

None.

Associated background

None.

Differential diagnosis

Indistinguishable from other types of macrophages.

Leydig cell

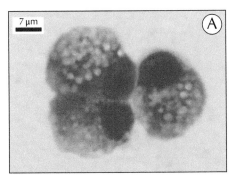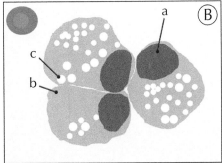

7 μm

Figure 70 - Photomicrograph (A) and schematic representation (B) of the Leydig cell.

General characteristics and biological function

Also known as 'interstitial cell'. In normal testis, these cells are located in the interstitium and are responsible for sex hormone (testosterone) production.

Shape and size

Medium-sized, pear-shaped cells with low nuclear:cytoplasmic ratio.

Nucleus

Round or ovoid, hyperchromatic, characterized by compact chromatin and localized at the cell periphery (a).

Cytoplasm

Abundant, moderately basophilic (b) and containing lipid vacuoles (c). In cats, lipid vacuoles are particularly abundant.

Location

Testicles.

Cytoarchitectures

Usually exfoliate as single cells; small aggregates forming perivascular cytoarchitecture are detectable.

Associated background

None.

Differential diagnosis

Macrophage (adipophage), sebocyte.

■ Lipoblast

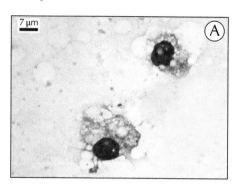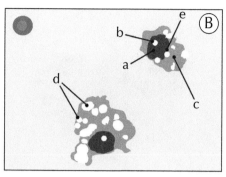

Figure 71 - Photomicrograph (A) and schematic representation (B) of the lipoblast.

General characteristics and biological function

Immature adipocyte. The lipoblast is also known as 'multilocular adipocyte'. It can be considered a mature form when part of brown fat.

Shape and size

Medium-sized cell, pleomorphic, with no well-defined cell boundaries and low nuclear:cytoplasmic ratio.

Nucleus

Round, peripheral (a), with compact chromatin and occasional optically empty vacuoles indenting the nucleus and/or possibly superimposed on the nucleus (b).

Cytoplasm

Abundant, moderately basophilic (c), occupied by large amount of round, variably sized, optically empty vacuoles (d), which in some cases indent the nucleus (e).

Location

Adipose tissue, immature adipose tissue, brown fat.

Cytoarchitectures

Large three-dimensional clusters together with mature adipocytes.

Associated background

Fat matrix.

Differential diagnosis

Adipophage, macrophage.

◼ Luteal cell

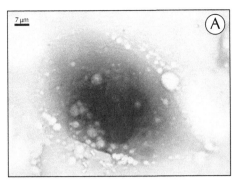
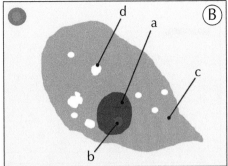

Figure 72 - Photomicrograph (A) and schematic representation (B) of the luteal cell.

General characteristics and biological function

Cell that forms the corpus luteum, producing progesterone.

Shape and size

Varies in size from very large (70–100 μm in major axis: 'macroluteocytes') to large (30–60 μm: 'microluteocytes'). Shape can be slightly pleomorphic, but mostly round or pear-shaped.

Nucleus

Large nucleus, round to oval, central to paracentral, characterized by finely stippled chromatin (a), with a prominent nucleolus (b).

Cytoplasm

Basophilic, abundant (c), with the presence of scattered, optically empty vacuoles (d).

Location

Female genital tract, ovary, corpus luteum.

Cytoarchitectures

These cells can form small pavement clusters, but are often distributed as single cells.

Associated background

None.

Differential diagnosis

None.

■ Lymphoglandular body

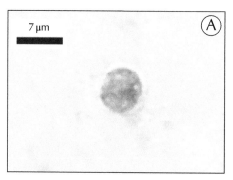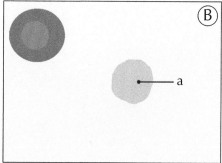

Figure 73 - Photomicrograph (A) and schematic representation (B) of the lymphoglandular body.

General characteristics and biological function

Cytoplasmic fragments resulting from the division of lymphoid cells in the context of lymphoid follicle activation.

Shape and size

Small and round, size ranging from approximately 5–7 μm (smaller than or comparable with erythrocyte).

Nucleus

Absent.

Cytoplasm

Basophilic (a).

Location

Lymph nodes and disseminated secondary follicles when hyperplastic/activated.

Cytoarchitectures

None.

Associated background

None.

Differential diagnosis

Platelet: lymphoglandular bodies are more basophilic and platelets are more eosinophilic. Polychromatophilic erythrocyte.

Macrophage

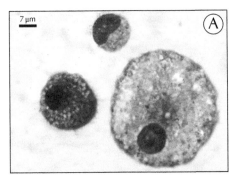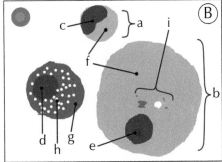

Figure 74 - Photomicrograph (A) and schematic representation (B) of the macrophage.

General characteristics and biological function

Cell derived from circulating monocyte which has migrated into the tissues and become a resident cell. Macrophage plays major roles in non-specific (phagocytosis) and specific (antigen-presenting cell) immunity. It is differently named based on the location in the body (liver: Kupffer cells; brain: microglia).

Shape and size

Highly variable from medium (a), to very large (b), and from round to pleomorphic in shape.

Nucleus

The nucleus is typically kidney-shaped (c) but can appear also round (d). It is consistently located in the peripheral or subterminal position. The chromatin appears finely stippled and a nucleolus can be detected occasionally (e).

Cytoplasm

The cytoplasm of the macrophage is characteristically rough, granular (f), amphophilic or moderately to strongly basophilic (g), and may contain optically empty vacuoles (h) or phagocytosed material which is usually no longer identifiable (i). It may also contain identifiable engulfed material. In some cases this latter feature is so pronounced that the cell is named after this (see Melanophage, Haemosiderophage).

Location

Reticuloendothelial system, many different tissues, areas of inflammation.

Cytoarchitectures

None in general. In special cases, it may be observed forming palisade clusters (see Epithelioid macrophage).

Associated background

None.

Differential diagnosis

Secreting cells, such as mammary foam cell, salivary gland cell, sebocyte.

■ Mammary foam cell

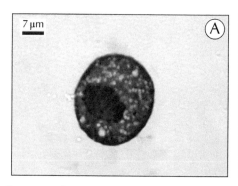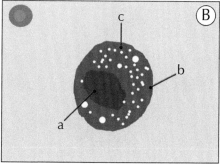

Figure 75 - Photomicrograph (A) and schematic representation (B) of the mammary foam cell.

General characteristics and biological function

Actively secreting cell of mammary epithelium, morphologically similar to macrophage.

Shape and size

Round or ovoid cell, with low nuclear:cytoplasmic ratio.

Nucleus

Oval to round, predominantly subterminal (a); can be slightly indented by intracytoplasmic lipid secretory vacuoles.

Cytoplasm

Eosinophilic (b), rich in optically empty vacuoles (c).

Location

Secreting mammary gland.

Cytoarchitectures

Can form pavement or three-dimensional cytoarchitectures, but also exfoliate as single elements. Arranged in papillary cytoarchitectures in hyperplastic phenomena.

Associated background

Fat–proteinaceous background, typical of the lactating gland.

Differential diagnosis

Macrophage. Sometimes, it is very difficult, if not impossible, to differentiate these cells from resident macrophages in the mammary gland.

■ Mammary gland cell

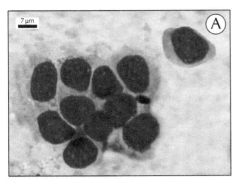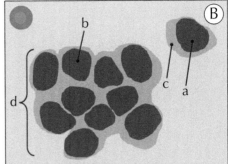

Figure 76 - Photomicrograph (A) and schematic representation (B) of the mammary gland cell.

General characteristics and biological function

Cells that form the epithelium of tubulo-alveolar structures of the mammary gland.

Shape and size

Small cells, cuboidal, with a intermediate–high nuclear:cytoplasmic ratio.

Nucleus

Oval to round, central (a) or polar (b), with coarse to clumped chromatin.

Cytoplasm

Weakly basophilic, smooth, with no particular detectable structures (c).

Location

Mammary gland.

Cytoarchitectures

Mammary cells primarily form pavement or trabecular clusters (d), or rarely acinar or tubular structures. In hyperplastic phenomena, papillary cytoarchitectures are detected.

Associated background

Proteinaceous and proteinaceous–fat background.

Differential diagnosis

Basal cell.

■ Mast cell

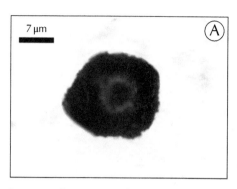 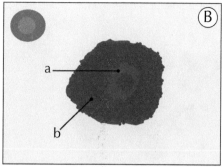

Figure 77 - Photomicrograph (A) and schematic representation (B) of the mast cell.

General characteristics and biological function

Mesenchymal cell localized within the connective tissue in different organs (stroma). Produces chemical mediators of inflammation.

Shape and size

Round to ovoid cell, medium-sized.

Nucleus

Central, sometimes difficult to see since it is obscured by the cytoplasmic granules (a).

Cytoplasm

Weakly eosinophilic, completely filled with magenta granules (b).

Location

Connective tissue support of various tissues and organs.

Cytoarchitectures

None.

Associated background

It is possible to find secretory granules in the background, where mast cells degranulated or ruptured during sample preparation.

Differential diagnosis

None.

Mature non-nucleated keratinized squamous cell

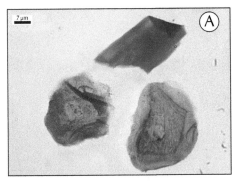 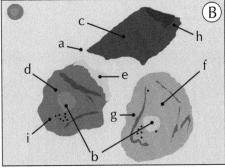

Figure 78 - Micrograph (A) and schematic representation (B) of the mature non-nucleated keratinized squamous cell.

General characteristics and biological function

Mature form of the process of keratinization in stratified squamous epithelia; also known as 'lamellar keratin' it represents what remains of the keratinized squamous epithelial cell, in its normal maturation process and exfoliation.

Shape and size

Large. The shape is clearly polygonal, with clear and unmistakable angles (a).

Nucleus

Absent, although in some cases it is possible to observe the area it previously occupied in the cell (b). This is sometimes referred to as a 'ghost cell'.

Cytoplasm

Abundant, it occupies the entire cell. The colour ranges from deep purple (c), to purple (d), to light blue (e), to grey (f). It may present numerous folds (g) and sometimes the cell folds back on itself (h). Small pigmentations can be detected (i).

Location

Surface keratinized epithelia.

Cytoarchitectures

Usually, in this stage of maturation these cells exfoliate individually because they lose the cohesive pattern of less mature stages.

Associated background

None.

Differential diagnosis

Adipocyte.

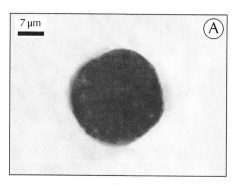
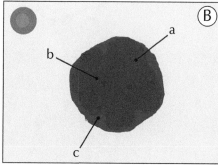

Figure 79 - Photomicrograph (A) and schematic representation (B) of the megakaryoblast.

General characteristics and biological function

Immature cell of the megakaryoblastic lineage, precursor of the promegakaryocyte.

Shape and size

Very large cell, round, with a high nuclear:cytoplasmic ratio.

Nucleus

Very large, with finely stippled chromatin, round to slightly multilobulated (a), with numerous nucleoli, sometimes visible (b). The nucleus will be subject to the phenomenon of 'endomytosis', which will give rise to polyploid multilobulated nucleus in the subsequent maturative stages.

Cytoplasm

Scant basophilic cytoplasm (c).

Location

Bone marrow.

Cytoarchitectures

None.

Associated background

None.

Differential diagnosis

Promegakaryocyte.

■ Megakaryocyte

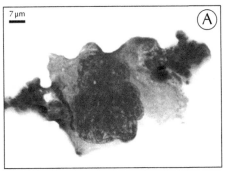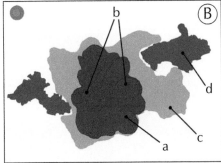

Figure 80 - Photomicrograph (A) and schematic representation (B) of the megakaryocyte.

General characteristics and biological function

Largest bone marrow cell producing circulating platelets by fragmentation of the cytoplasm.

Shape and size

Very large (40–100 μm in diameter), pleomorphic.

Nucleus

Large nucleus (a), characterized by several lobes (b), with rarely identifiable nucleoli.

Cytoplasm

Abundant and eosinophilic (c) if compared with that of promegakaryocyte and megakaryoblast.

Location

Bone marrow.

Cytoarchitectures

Can be associated with platelets (d).

Associated background

None.

Differential diagnosis

Other giant cells: osteoblast, inflammatory giant cell, megakaryoblast and promegakaryocyte.

■ Melanocyte

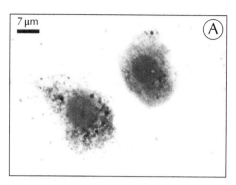
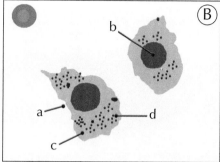

Figure 81 - Photomicrograph (A) and schematic representation (B) of the melanocyte.

General characteristics and biological function

Melanin-producing cell associated with epidermis, mucosae and, more rarely, serosal surfaces.

Shape and size

Medium-sized, with pleomorphic morphology, with no defined cellular limits (a).

Nucleus

Large, round, central, with fine to finely stippled chromatin (b).

Cytoplasm

Abundant, faintly basophilic (c), occupied by large numbers of fine, dark melanin granules (d).

Location

Pigmented areas of the body.

Cytoarchitectures

None.

Associated background

Free melanin pigment can be evident in the background.

Differential diagnosis

Melanophage.

■ Melanophage

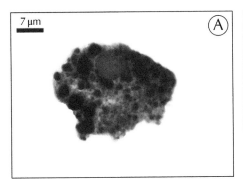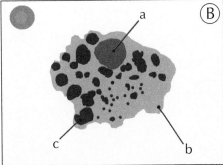

Figure 82 - Photomicrograph (A) and schematic representation (B) of the melanophage.

General characteristics and biological function

Macrophage phagocytosing excess melanin.

Shape and size

See Macrophage.

Nucleus

See Macrophage (a).

Cytoplasm

See Macrophage (b). Variably sized, dark brown, coarse aggregates (melanin) are evident in the cytoplasm (c). The aggregates are larger and more irregular than those in the melanocyte.

Location

Locations with high production of melanin.

Cytoarchitectures

None.

Associated background

Free melanin pigment can be evident in the background.

Differential diagnosis

Melanocyte; macrophages containing different pigments.

■ Mesothelial cell

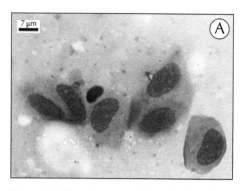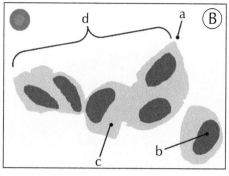

Figure 83 - Photomicrograph (A) and schematic representation (B) of the mesothelial cell.

General characteristics and biological function

Cell lining serous cavities. The morphology of these cells changes considerably when involved in inflammation (see Activated mesothelial cell).

Shape and size

Medium-sized cell with squamous-like appearance, with pronounced corners (a), polygonal in shape.

Nucleus

Ovoid, with fine to finely stippled chromatin (b).

Cytoplasm

Amphophilic and smooth without particular intracytoplasmic structures (c). The cytoplasm is thin which gives a flattened appearance to the cell.

Location

Serous cavities.

Cytoarchitectures

Pavement cytoarchitectures (d).

Associated background

None.

Differential diagnosis

Endotheliocyte if not forming typical capillary structures. Epithelial cells.

■ Metamyelocyte

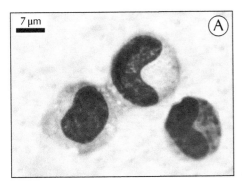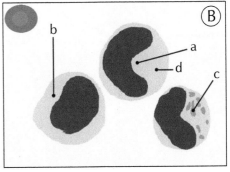

Figure 84 - Photomicrograph (A) and schematic representation (B) of the metamyelocyte.

General characteristics and biological function

Myeloid cell, intermediate form between myelocyte and band cell cytotypes.

Shape and size

Round cell, discrete, medium in size.

Nucleus

Characteristic kidney-shaped (a), with finely granular but not clearly condensed chromatin (less condensed compared to the band cell).

Cytoplasm

The cytoplasm is clear (b). It may characterized by typical granules of eosinophil (c) or basophil lineages, or, in the case of neutrophil precursor, the granules are not visible (d).

Location

Bone marrow.

Cytoarchitectures

None.

Associated background

None.

Differential diagnosis

Band cell.

■ Metarubricyte

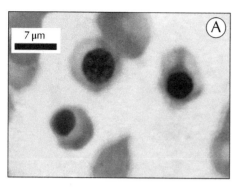
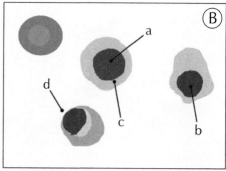

Figure 85 - Photomicrograph (A) and schematic representation (B) of the metarubricyte.

General characteristics and biological function

Last stage of nucleated red blood cell maturation. It follows the stage of rubricyte and precedes the stage of polychromatophilic erythrocyte.

Shape and size

Small cell, round, sometimes elongated.

Nucleus

The nucleus presents with highly clumped chromatin (a) or may be pyknotic (b), central (c), or in the process of being expelled from the cell (d).

Cytoplasm

Eosinophilic or similar to erythrocyte cytoplasm.

Location

Bone marrow.

Cytoarchitectures

None.

Associated background

None.

Differential diagnosis

Small lymphocyte.

■ Microorganism-laden macrophage

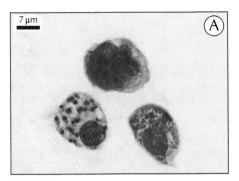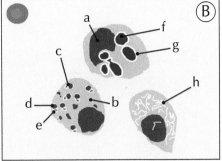

Figure 86 - Photomicrograph (A) and schematic representation (B) of the microorganism-laden macrophage.

General characteristics and biological function

Macrophage actively engaged in phagocytosis of microorganisms.

Shape and size

See Macrophage.

Nucleus

See Macrophage (a).

Cytoplasm

See Macrophage (b). Inside the cytoplasm there are engulfed microorganisms. Typical examples: protozoa – *Leishmania* spp. (c), characterized by the nucleus (d) and kinetoplast (e); fungi – *Cryptococcus* spp. (f), characterized by colourless capsule (g); bacteria – mycobacteria (h), characterized by the absence of staining (negative image).

Location

Sites of protozoal, fungal or bacterial infection.

Cytoarchitectures

None.

Associated background

None.

Differential diagnosis

None.

■ Monoblast

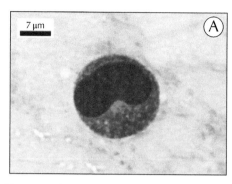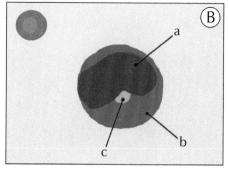

Figure 87 - Photomicrograph (A) and schematic representation (B) of the monoblast.

General characteristics and biological function

Bone marrow precursor of monocytes.

Shape and size

Large round cell.

Nucleus

Round, irregular or kidney-shaped, with finely stippled chromatin (a) (precursors of granulocytes have more coarse chromatin pattern in comparison), with occasional presence of one or more visible nucleoli.

Cytoplasm

Basophilic (b), characterized by the perinuclear Golgi area, often located close to the nuclear indentation (c).

Location

Bone marrow.

Cytoarchitectures

None.

Associated background

None.

Differential diagnosis

Myelocytes and precursors of the granulocytic line; often it is really difficult to differentiate them.

■ Monocyte

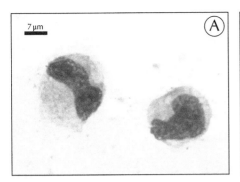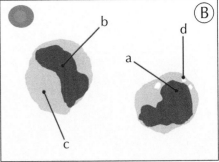

Figure 88 - Photomicrograph (A) and schematic representation (B) of the monocyte.

General characteristics and biological function

Circulating cell, the precursor of tissue macrophages.

Shape and size

The largest circulating cell, from round to pleomorphic.

Nucleus

Variable in shape, with irregular or pleated outline (a), 'horseshoe' or bilobed (b), with finely stippled chromatin.

Cytoplasm

Abundant, moderately basophilic, blue (c), rough, may contain some vacuoles (d).

Location

Circulating blood, bone marrow.

Cytoarchitectures

None.

Associated background

None.

Differential diagnosis

Macrophage.

■ Mott cell

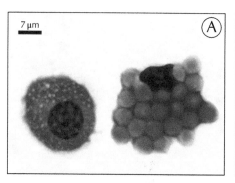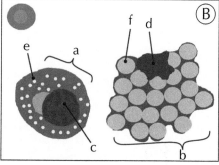

Figure 89 - Photomicrograph (A; Source: Courtesy of Carlo Masserdotti) and schematic representation (B) of the Mott cell.

General characteristics and biological function

Particular type of plasma cell containing characteristic cytoplasmic inclusions known as 'Russell bodies'.

Shape and size

The morphology of the Mott cell ranges from being comparable to the traditional plasma cell (a), to a typical 'grape' morphology (b), depending on the size of the inclusions.

Nucleus

May be similar to that of the plasma cell (c) or localized in the periphery and indented (d) by the inclusions.

Cytoplasm

Characterized by intracytoplasmic pale pink inclusions ('Russell bodies'), ranging from punctate/small (e) to large (f), which can also occupy the entire cytoplasm area.

Location

Lymph nodes and sites characterized by particularly strong production of immuno-globulins, including areas of chronic inflammation.

Cytoarchitectures

None.

Associated background

None.

Differential diagnosis

In the case of 'grape' morphology, these cells may be confused with macrophages and sebocytes.

◼ Myeloblast

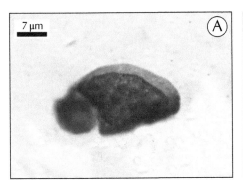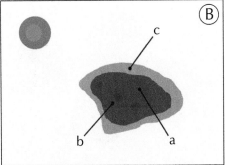

Figure 90 - Photomicrograph (A) and schematic representation (B) of the myeloblast.

General characteristics and biological function

Most immature myeloid progenitor cell. It precedes the promyelocyte stage.

Shape and size

Spheroidal or ovoid, but also slightly irregular, smaller than promyelocyte with higher nuclear:cytoplasmic ratio.

Nucleus

Fine chromatin, spheroidal or polygonal (a), with one to five visible nucleoli (b).

Cytoplasm

Basophilic, scant, with no visible granules (c).

Location

Bone marrow.

Cytoarchitectures

None.

Associated background

None.

Differential diagnosis

Promyelocyte, immature lymphoid cell (e.g. centroblast).

■ Myelocyte

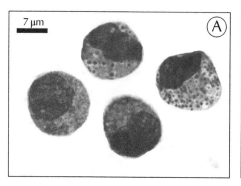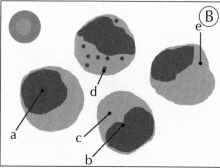

Figure 91 - Photomicrograph (A) and schematic representation (B) of the myelocyte.

General characteristics and biological function

Maturing granulocyte cell of the myeloid lineage. It follows the stage of promyelo-cyte and precedes the metamyelocyte.

Shape and size

Round, large cell, smaller than promyelocyte.

Nucleus

Spheroidal (a) or slightly indented (b), located in a peripheral position, with finely stippled to lacy chromatin and no clearly visible nucleoli.

Cytoplasm

Slightly basophilic. Contains specific and azurophilic granules, which are not visi-ble, in the case of neutrophil precursor (c). Granules are identifiable in the case of basophil (d) and eosinophil (e) precursor.

Location

Bone marrow.

Cytoarchitectures

None.

Associated background

None.

Differential diagnosis

Promyelocyte.

■ Myoepithelial cell

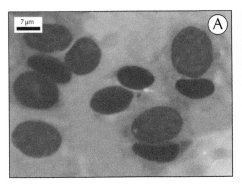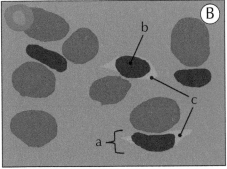

Figure 92 - Photomicrograph (A) and schematic representation (B) of the myoepithelial cell.

General characteristics and biological function

Cells located between the secretory cells and the basement membrane in apocrine glands. They are characterized by both contractile (mesenchymal) and epithelial features.

Shape and size

Fusiform cell. When exfoliates is identifiable from its elongated morphology (a), associated with apocrine epithelial cells.

Nucleus

The nuclei appear ovoid to spindle-shaped, hyperchromatic, with dense chromatin (b).

Cytoplasm

Scant, bipolar and weakly basophilic (c).

Location

Basal portion of apocrine and modified apocrine glands.

Cytoarchitectures

Associated with typical cytoarchitectures formed by different apocrine or modified apocrine cells.

Associated background

None.

Differential diagnosis

If isolated, it is not possible to differentiate myoepithelial cells from other types of spindle cells (e.g. smooth muscle cell, fibrocyte).

■ Neuron

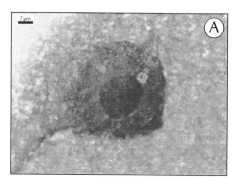 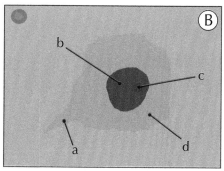

Figure 93 - Micrograph (A) and schematic representation (B) of the neuron.

General characteristics and biological function

Neural cell responsible for transmission of, processing and receiving nerve impulses.

Shape and size

Very large cell, round, stellate, or pear-shaped, with a low nuclear:cytoplasmic ratio. A peripheral cone-shaped area is often evident (a).

Nucleus

Central, ovoid or round (b). Finely reticular chromatin, with a large nucleolus (c).

Cytoplasm

Basophilic and abundant (d), granular, without particular structures.

Location

Central nervous system and ganglia.

Cytoarchitectures

None.

Associated background

Granular proteinaceous matrix.

Differential diagnosis

None.

■ Neutrophil

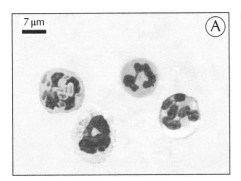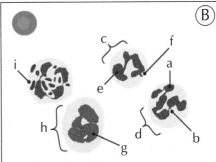

Figure 94 - Photomicrograph (A) and schematic representation (B) of the neutrophil.

General characteristics and biological function

Circulating granulocyte which represents the first line of defence in inflammation.

Shape and size

Round cell, 12–15 µm in diameter.

Nucleus

Characteristically segmented into multiple (three to five) lobulations (a), the number of which is directly proportional to the cell's age. Lobulations are joined by thin segments of chromatin (b). Younger cells have relatively few lobulations (c) if compared with older ones (d). The chromatin is compact to clumped (e). In female subjects it is sometimes possible to identify a very small 'clubbed' protrusion, which represents the chromatin of the Barr body (f). When they exude in tissues (inflammation), the morphology of the nucleus soon changes, becoming less lobulated, discoloured and distended due to the influx of fluids (g). This particular appearance is referred to as 'degenerate neutrophil' (h).

Cytoplasm

Light, moderately granular, rich in granules (azurophilic and specific) which have weak affinity for commonly used stains (from which derives the name 'neutrophil'). It is possible to find engulfed microorganisms inside the neutrophil cytoplasm (i) during bacterial infection.

Location

Circulating blood, bone marrow, tissues with inflammation and infection.

Cytoarchitectures

None.

Associated background

None.

Differential diagnosis

Basophil, band cell.

■ Non-keratinized squamous epithelial cell

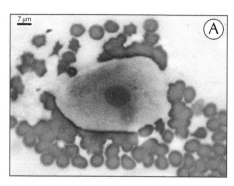 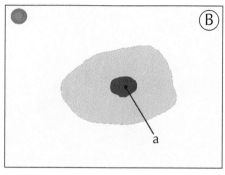

Figure 95 - Photomicrograph (A) and schematic representation (B) of the non-keratinized squamous epithelial cell.

General characteristics and biological function

Epithelial cell lining body surfaces (mucosae) covered by stratified epithelia that does not keratinize. Also represents the maturational stage antecedent to the keratinized squamous epithelial cell in those areas (e.g. epidermis) characterized by keratinization.

Shape and size

Flattened cell, with low nuclear:cytoplasmic ratio; thin resembling a 'scale', with polygonal morphology (with angular less marked angular edges compared with keratinized squamous epithelial cell) and evident cell limits.

Nucleus

Central (a), with finely stippled compact chromatin, or pyknotic appearance.

Cytoplasm

Abundant, smooth, with no particular structures.

Location

Outermost layer of non-keratinized epithelia (e.g. mucosae), or superficial layers of keratinized epithelia.

Cytoarchitectures

These cells exfoliate as single cells or grouped in small pavement clusters.

Associated background

None.

Differential diagnosis

Intermediate squamous epithelial cell.

■ Normochromatic rubricyte

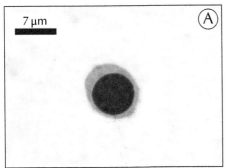 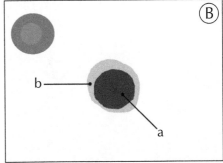

7 µm

Figure 96 - Micrograph (A), and schematic representation (B) of the normochromatic rubricyte.

General characteristics and biological function

Erythropoietic cell, maturing from polychromatic rubricyte to metarubricyte. It represents the last maturation stage of rubricytes.

Shape and size

Small cell, discrete, round, with high nuclear:cytoplasmic ratio.

Nucleus

Round, central (a), with compact chromatin.

Cytoplasm

Scant, pinkish-grey, very similar to erythrocyte cytoplasm (b).

Location

Bone marrow.

Cytoarchitectures

None.

Associated background

None.

Differential diagnosis

Small lymphocytes, metarubricyte, other rubricyte stages.

■ Oligodendrocyte

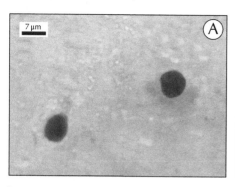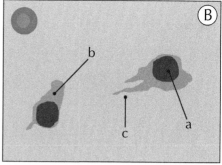

Figure 97 - Micrograph (A) and schematic representation (B) of the oligodendrocyte.

General characteristics and biological function

Cell responsible for myelin production and nerve support in the central nervous system.

Shape and size

Small cell, with poorly defined cytoplasmic limits.

Nucleus

Small, round with compact chromatin (a).

Cytoplasm

Scant, weakly basophilic (b), whose often subtle prolongations (c) are not easily identified.

Location

Central nervous system.

Cytoarchitectures

None.

Associated background

Granular proteinaceous matrix.

Differential diagnosis

Small lymphocyte.

■ Oocyte

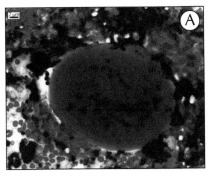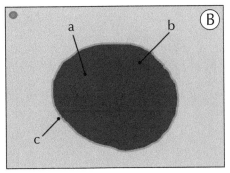

Figure 98 - Micrograph (A) and schematic representation (B) of the oocyte.

General characteristics and biological function

The largest cell in the body, the female gamete.

Shape and size

Very large size, typically round or 'rugby ball' shaped.

Nucleus

Very large. It is not always possible to identify it due to the hyperbasophilic cytoplasm (a).

Cytoplasm

Abundant and hyperbasophilic (b). It has a marginal zone, the 'zona pellucida' which is particularly smooth in appearance (c).

Location

Female genital tract, ovary.

Cytoarchitectures

None.

Associated background

None.

Differential diagnosis

None.

■ Osteoblast

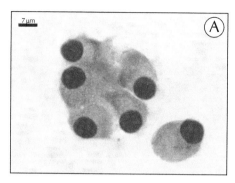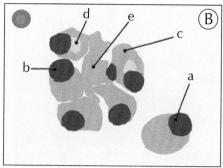

Figure 99 - Micrograph (A) and schematic representation (B) of the osteoblast.

General characteristics and biological function

Mesenchymal cell producing osteoid in bone tissue.

Shape and size

Large, ovoid to pear-shaped, with a low nuclear:cytoplasmic ratio. Despite being mesenchymal, it may resemble a discrete cell.

Nucleus

Typically round and apparently positioned slightly outside ('punched out') of the cell outline (a). Often a single large nucleolus is evident (b).

Cytoplasm

Abundant, basophilic (c), often with evident clear perinuclear Golgi area (d).

Location

Skeletal system, bone tissue.

Cytoarchitectures

Sometimes, osteoblasts can be found clustered around osteoid matrix, but, due to their shape, it is not a typical storiform cytoarchitecture.

Associated background

Osteoid matrix (e).

Differential diagnosis

Plasma cells.

■ Osteoclast

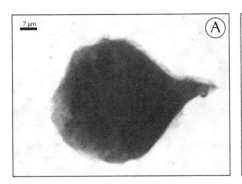
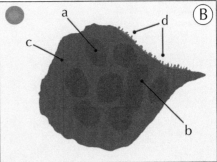

Figure 100 - Micrograph (A) and schematic representation (B) of the osteoclast.

General characteristics and biological function

Multinucleated cell of myeloid origin responsible for bone resorption.

Shape and size

Pleomorphic or ovoid, very large cell.

Nucleus

These cells contain eight to 15 nuclei of ovoid shape (a), which are homogeneous in size and shape and haphazardly arranged. Some nucleoli may be prominent (b).

Cytoplasm

Intensely basophilic (c), with a corrugated eosinophilic edge (d), made up of folds of the cytoplasm, which represent the areas of the interface with the mineralized bone: ripples in this area are concentrate acids used for bone lysis.

Location

Skeletal system, bone tissue.

Cytoarchitectures

None.

Associated background

None or osteoid matrix.

Differential diagnosis

Inflammatory giant cell, megakaryocyte, promegakaryocyte.

■ Parabasal squamous epithelial cell

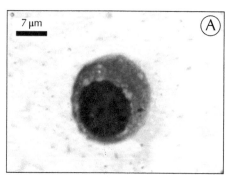
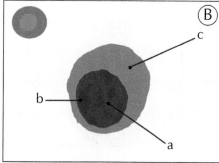

Figure 101 - Photomicrograph (A) and schematic representation (B) of the parabasal squamous epithelial cell.

General characteristics and biological function

Epithelial lining cell of stratified epithelia of intermediate morphology between basal cell and intermediate squamous epithelial cell.

Shape and size

Cells of intermediate size, round to ovoid, with intermediate nuclear:cytoplasmic ratio, lower than that of basal cell.

Nucleus

Central or subterminal, large (a), with coarse to finely stippled chromatin (b).

Cytoplasm

Basophilic, it occupies about half of the surface of the cell (c), with some occasional perinuclear vacuolation.

Location

Epithelia. In particular, this cell type from vaginal epithelium is important in assessment of cycle phases.

Cytoarchitectures

Found as individual cells or forms pavement cytoarchitectures.

Associated background

None.

Differential diagnosis

Macrophages, basal cells.

■ Parathyroid chief cell

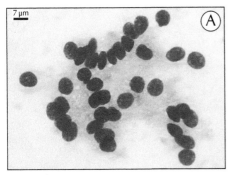
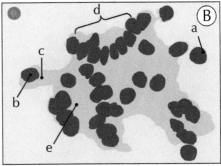

Figure 102 - Micrograph (A; Source: Courtesy of Carlo Masserdotti) and schematic representation (B) of the parathyroid chief cell.

General characteristics and biological function

Endocrine cell forming the parenchyma of the parathyroid gland, responsible for the production of parathyroid hormone.

Shape and size

Medium-sized cell, characterized by faded margins which are difficult to detect. Often appears as 'naked nucleus' (a).

Nucleus

Round (b) or slightly ovoid, with finely stippled chromatin, without evident nucleoli, or, when detectable, of small size.

Cytoplasm

Mildly basophilic, blue, with moderately granular texture (c), whose boundaries are not easy to detect.

Location

Parathyroid gland.

Cytoarchitectures

These cells may form palisade (d) or more rarely acinar-like (rosette (e)) cytoarchitectures.

Associated background

None.

Differential diagnosis

Other endocrine cells: adrenal cell, parathyroid chief cell

■ Pituicyte

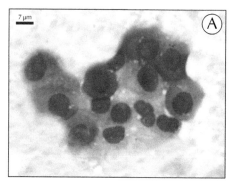 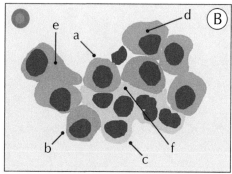

Figure 103 - Photomicrograph (A) and schematic representation (B) of the pituicyte.

General characteristics and biological function

Endocrine cells which secrete different hormones. Acidophilic cells (a): growth hormone and prolactin; basophilic cells (b): thyrotropic hormone, gonadotropin and adrenocorticotropic hormone; chromophobe cells (c) are considered to be resting cells.

Shape and size

Acidophilic (a) and basophilic (b): round/oval, medium-sized. Chromophobe (c): smaller and rounder than acidophilic and basophilic cells.

Nucleus

From round to oval, occasionally indented.

Cytoplasm

Acidophilic cell: orange (d); basophilic cell: blue (e); chromophobe: grey (f).

Location

Adenohypophysis.

Cytoarchitectures

Tend to exfoliate in pavement/three-dimensional clusters, or form perivascular cyto-architectures, containing all three cell types.

Associated background

Possible blood from the abundant vascularization of the gland.

Differential diagnosis

None.

Plasma cell

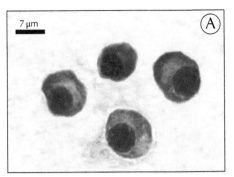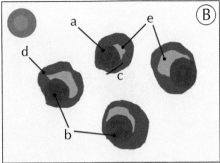

Figure 104 - Micrograph (A) and schematic representation (B) of the plasma cell.

General characteristics and biological function

Lymphoid cell differentiated for the production of antibodies. Originates from the immunoblast through the plasmacytoid cell stage.

Shape and size

Discrete cell, intermediate in size, ovoid shape.

Nucleus

Round, located in subterminal position (a), the chromatin is characterized by the presence of large clumps (b), which determine the 'clockface' appearance (c) consistently evident in histology, but not always identifiable in cytology.

Cytoplasm

Strongly basophilic (d), characterized by the presence of a large clear perinuclear area (e), which represents the Golgi apparatus.

Location

Lymph nodes, bone marrow; locations of chronic inflammation with a prominent B cell immune response.

Cytoarchitectures

None.

Associated background

None.

Differential diagnosis

Osteoblast, plasmacytoid cells.

■ Plasmacytoid cell

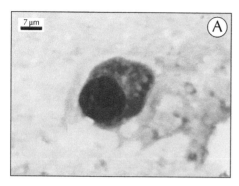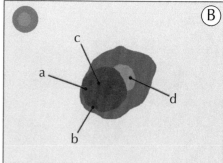

Figure 105 - Photomicrograph (A) and schematic representation (B) of the plasmacytoid cell.

General characteristics and biological function

Also called 'plasmablast', is a lymphoid cell transforming from the immunoblast stage to that of plasma cell. It contains intermediate characters between the two cell types.

Shape and size

Medium-sized to large cells, oval in shape.

Nucleus

The nucleus is large, round and is located paracentrally (a). Contains some chromatin clusters (b) and the nucleolus is visible (c).

Cytoplasm

Intensely basophilic with clear perinuclear Golgi area (d).

Location

Active lymph nodes and tissue-associated lymphoid follicles.

Cytoarchitectures

None.

Associated background

None.

Differential diagnosis

Immunoblast, plasma cell.

■ Platelet

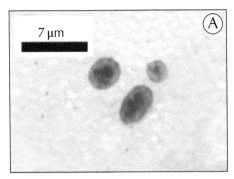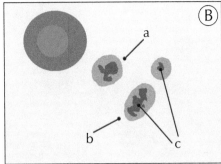

Figure 106 - Micrograph (A) and schematic representation (B) of the platelet.

General characteristics and biological function

Platelets are derived from segmentation of cytoplasmic processes of megakaryocytes. They are found isolated, but also in small aggregates, and are involved in coagulation.

Shape and size

Round (a) to ovoid–elongated (b).

Nucleus

Absent.

Cytoplasm

Dotted with small to medium-sized pink granules (c). Often there is a certain degree of physiological anisocytosis between platelets of the same subject.

Location

Circulating blood.

Cytoarchitectures

Platelets can form small pavement or three-dimensional cytoarchitectures when coagulation is activated.

Associated background

None.

Differential diagnosis

Lymphoglandular body.

■ Pneumocyte

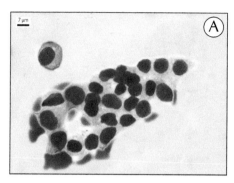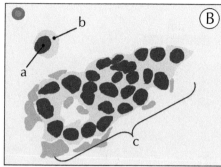

Figure 107 - Photomicrograph (A) and schematic representation (B) of the pneumocyte.

General characteristics and biological function

The pneumocytes are epithelial cells that form the lining of the alveoli. There are two types (I and II).

Shape and size

It is not possible to morphologically differentiate the two types of pneumocyte. The cells are small in size, with intermediate nuclear:cytoplasmic ratio and a generally round shape.

Nucleus

Central, protruding ('bullseye' morphology), large, with compact chromatin (a).

Cytoplasm

Abundant cytoplasm, smooth, with no particular detectable internal structures (b).

Location

Pulmonary alveoli.

Cytoarchitectures

Typically organized in pavement cytoarchitectures (c).

Associated background

None.

Differential diagnosis

Alveolar macrophage if not particularly activated.

■ Polychromatic rubricyte

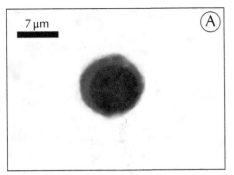
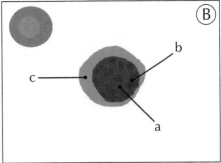

Figure 108 - Micrograph (A) and schematic representation (B) of the polychromatic rubricyte.

General characteristics and biological function

Erythropoietic cell, maturing from basophilic rubricyte into normochromatic rubricyte. It represents the second/intermediate maturation stage of rubricytes.

Shape and size

Small cell, discrete, round, with a high nuclear:cytoplasmic ratio.

Nucleus

Round, central (a), with chromatin clumped in large clusters (b).

Cytoplasm

Grey–blue/purple (less basophilic than basophilic rubricyte), scant (c).

Location

Bone marrow.

Cytoarchitectures

None.

Associated background

None.

Differential diagnosis

Small lymphocyte, prorubricyte, other rubricyte stages.

■ Polychromatophilic erythrocyte

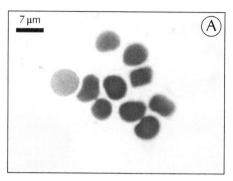 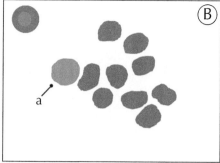

Figure 109 - Photomicrograph (A) and schematic representation (B) of the polychromatophilic erythrocyte.

General characteristics and biological function

Also known as 'reticulocyte', represents the young stage of the erythrocyte, immediately after the metarubricyte stage.

Shape and size

Non-nucleated cell, round, larger than mature erythrocyte (a).

Nucleus

Absent.

Cytoplasm

Very pale basophilic, bluer than erythrocyte.

Location

Bone marrow, sometimes circulating blood.

Associated background

None.

Differential diagnosis

Erythrocyte, lymphoglandular body.

■ Promegakaryocyte

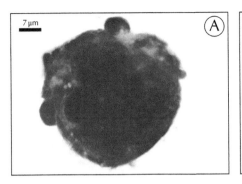 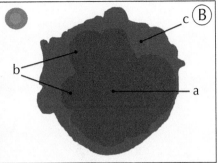

Figure 110 - Micrograph (A) and schematic representation (B) of the promegakaryocyte.

General characteristics and biological function

Large bone marrow cell, maturation stage between megakaryoblast and megakaryocyte.

Shape and size

Large cell, with a high nuclear:cytoplasmic ratio.

Nucleus

Large, multilobed (a) – two to four lobulations (b).

Cytoplasm

Moderate amount of cytoplasm (more abundant than in megakaryoblast), and basophilic (less so than in megakaryoblast) (c).

Location

Bone marrow.

Cytoarchitectures

None.

Associated background

None.

Differential diagnosis

Megakaryoblast, osteoclast, megakaryocyte.

CYTOTYPES

■ Promyelocyte

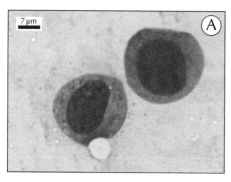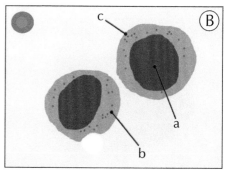

Figure 111 - Micrograph (A) and schematic representation (B) of the promyelocyte.

General characteristics and biological function

Myeloid cell that follows myeloblast and precedes myelocyte in the maturation of granulocyte.

Shape and size

Largest cell of the granulocytic cell line, larger than the myeloblast, although it is the following maturational step. Nuclear:cytoplasmic ratio is intermediate.

Nucleus

The nucleus (a) is round or ovoid–elongated, similar to that of myeloblasts. The chromatin is finely stippled and nucleoli are not always detectable.

Cytoplasm

Basophilic (b), less basophilic than that of myeloblasts, with barely visible small pink granules (c).

Location

Bone marrow.

Cytoarchitectures

None.

Associated background

None.

Differential diagnosis

Myeloblast, myelocyte.

■ Prorubricyte

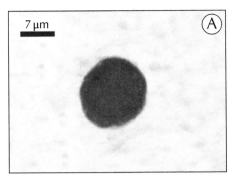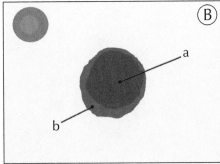

Figure 112 - Micrograph (A) and schematic representation (B) of the prorubricyte.

General characteristics and biological function

Bone marrow cell that originates from rubriblast and differentiates into rubricyte.

Shape and size

Cell with high nuclear:cytoplasmic ratio, round in shape.

Nucleus

Round, central or slightly eccentric, with fine chromatin and no prominent nucleoli (a).

Cytoplasm

Basophilic (may be less basophilic than rubriblast), scant (b).

Location

Bone marrow.

Cytoarchitectures

None.

Associated background

None.

Differential diagnosis

Rubriblast, centroblast.

■ Prostate cell

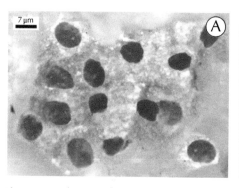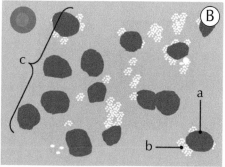

Figure 113 - Photomicrograph (A; Source: Courtesy of Carlo Masserdotti) and schematic representation (B) of the prostate cell.

General characteristics and biological function

Secreting cells of the prostate gland. They produce prostatic fluid essential for ejaculation.

Shape and size

Cuboidal to polygonal cells, small, with low nuclear:cytoplasmic ratio.

Nucleus

Round or ovoid, with compact chromatin, predominantly central (a).

Cytoplasm

Finely vacuolated with a dusty appearance (b); this feature is conferred by the secretory granules, which are very fine.

Location

Male reproductive system, prostate gland.

Cytoarchitectures

These cells typically exfoliate in honeycomb cytoarchitectures (c).

Associated background

None.

Differential diagnosis

Macrophage.

■ Renal tubular cell

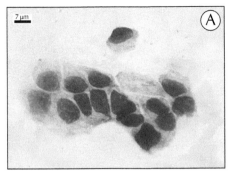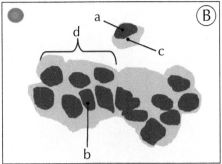

Figure 114 - Photomicrograph (A) and schematic representation (B) of the renal tubular cell.

General characteristics and biological function

Epithelial cell of the kidney tubules. Involved in solute balance regulation and detoxification.

Shape and size

Intermediate size, basically cuboidal shape, with intermediate nuclear:cytoplasmic ratio.

Nucleus

Round (a), sometimes cuboidal (b), peripheral position, with finely to finely stippled chromatin; usually nucleoli are not prominent.

Cytoplasm

Occupies about half of the area of the cell (c); moderately basophilic, without particular structures detectable.

Location

Cortex and medulla of kidney.

Cytoarchitectures

Tubular (d).

Associated background

None.

Differential diagnosis

None.

■ Rhabdomyocyte

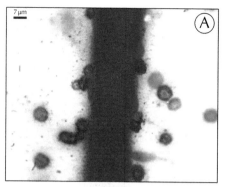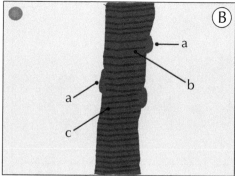

Figure 115 - Photomicrograph (A) and schematic representation (B) of the rhabdomyocyte.

General characteristics and biological function

Multinucleated contractile voluntary cell. Responsible for contraction of skeletal muscles.

Shape and size

Syncytium of cells, cylindrical in shape, diameter 10–100 μm and up to several centimetres in length. They are often detectable in cytological preparations as cell fragments.

Nucleus

Elongated/ovoid nuclei localized at the periphery (a) of the cell.

Cytoplasm

Basophilic (b) with densely cluttered basophilic myofibrils characterized by typical transverse bands (c).

Location

Musculoskeletal system, skeletal muscles.

Associated background

None.

Differential diagnosis

Cardiomyocyte.

◼ Rubriblast

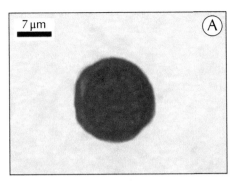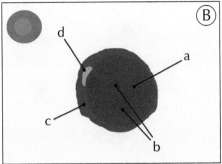

Figure 116 - Micrograph (A) and schematic representation (B) of the rubriblast.

General characteristics and biological function

The most immature progenitor cell of the erythroid lineage. The prorubricyte is derived from this cytotype.

Shape and size

The largest cell of the erythroid lineage, round, with a high nuclear:cytoplasmic ratio.

Nucleus

Characterized by finely stippled chromatin (a), and by one to three visible nucleoli (b).

Cytoplasm

Scant, intensely basophilic, deep blue (c), homogeneous, with no observable structures, except for the occasional presence of the perinuclear Golgi area (d).

Location

Bone marrow.

Cytoarchitectures

None.

Associated background

None.

Differential diagnosis

Immunoblast, centroblast.

■ Salivary gland cell

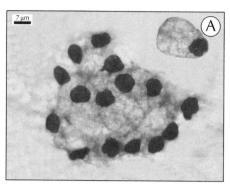 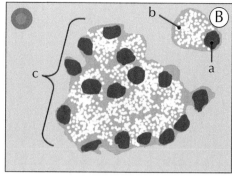

Figure 117 - Photomicrograph (A; Source: Courtesy of Carlo Masserdotti) and schematic representation (B) of the salivary gland cell.

General characteristics and biological function

Epithelial cells responsible for secreting saliva.

Shape and size

Medium-sized cells, pear-shaped, with low nuclear:cytoplasmic ratio.

Nucleus

Small and round, peripheral, characterized by compact chromatin (a).

Cytoplasm

Richly microvacuolated, with foamy appearance (b).

Location

Major salivary glands.

Cytoarchitectures

Typically exfoliate in a pavement cluster (c), or sometimes in three-dimensional clusters.

Associated background

None or proteinaceous.

Differential diagnosis

Macrophage, adipophage, sebocyte.

■ Sebocyte

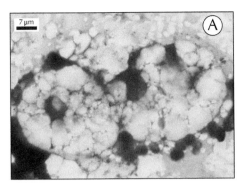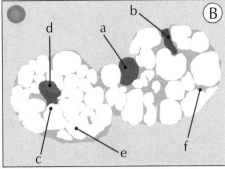

Figure 118 - Photomicrograph (A; Source: Courtesy of Carlo Masserdotti) and schematic representation (B) of the sebocyte.

General characteristics and biological function

Cell of the sebaceous glands producing sebum via olocrine secretion.

Shape and size

Medium to large in size, round to polygonal, with low nuclear:cytoplasmic ratio.

Nucleus

Peripheral to subterminal, from round (a) to flattened/crushed (b) due to the pressure of the secretion vacuoles. Often indentations (c) are evident as well as vacuoles that overlap the nucleus (d). Compact chromatin.

Cytoplasm

Cluttered by empty vacuoles which are round or polygonal in shape and very variable in size (e). In cats, the vacuoles are more homogeneous, small and regular compared to those in the dog. The cytoplasm is difficult to detect: it is observed only in small areas in between vacuoles (f).

Location

Dermis, sebaceous glands.

Cytoarchitectures

Almost always form three-dimensional cytoarchitectures.

Associated background

Fat matrix.

Differential diagnosis

Adipophage, lipoblast.

■ Sertoli cell

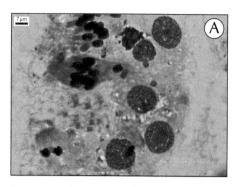 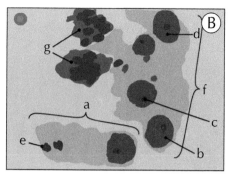

Figure 119 - Photomicrograph (A) and schematic representation (B) of the Sertoli cell.

General characteristics and biological function

Also known as 'nurse cell', has trophic function for sperm in the seminiferous tubules of the male genitalia and produces some hormones, including oestrogens.

Shape and size

Very large cells (a), elongated, irregular margins and low nuclear:cytoplasmic ratio.

Nucleus

Located in the basal zone, oval (b), with a visible nucleolus (c) and reticular chromatin (d).

Cytoplasm

Slightly basophilic, containing small granules. Nuclei of developing spermatogenic cells are often recognized within the cytoplasm or overlapping folds (e).

Location

Male genitalia, testis.

Cytoarchitectures

Often form a palisade (f), in association with group of developing spermatogenic cells (g).

Associated background

Often proteinaceous material with spermatozoa.

Differential diagnosis

Epididymal cells: lack of stereocilia is a feature.

■ Small lymphocyte

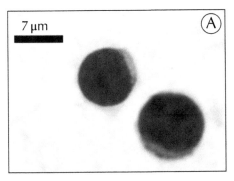
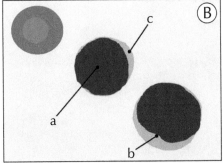

Figure 120 - Micrograph (A) and schematic representation (B) of the small lymphocyte.

General characteristics and biological function

Circulating cell and also colonizes lymphoid organs. Primarily involved in immune surveillance. The small lymphocyte morphology represents both B and T phenotypes (they are not identifiable morphologically). Either before (naïve) or after stimulation and clonal expansion (committed and/or memory).

Shape and size

Approximately 9 µm, round, with high nuclear:cytoplasmic ratio.

Nucleus

Round (a), central to paracentral, sometimes slightly indented (b), with compact chromatin. Rarely large chromatin aggregates are detected.

Cytoplasm

Scant, when visible, mainly at one cell pole (c).

Location

Circulating blood, parenchyma of the lymphoid organs and tissue-associated lymphatic nodules. Detected at sites of chronic inflammation.

Cytoarchitectures

None.

Associated background

None.

Differential diagnosis

Basal cell, centrocyte, metarubricyte.

■ Smooth muscle cell

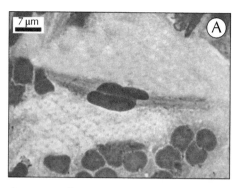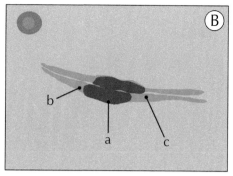

Figure 121 - Photomicrograph (A) and schematic representation (B) of the smooth muscle cell.

General characteristics and biological function

Mesenchymal cell responsible for involuntary contraction of many different tissues and organs.

Shape and size

Elongated thin cell, approximately 5 µm in diameter.

Nucleus

Elongated and thin (a), typically with blunt ends (b) which gives a cigar-shaped appearance.

Cytoplasm

Eosinophilic (c), with no identifiable structures.

Location

Involuntary muscle tissue of many viscera and vessels.

Cytoarchitectures

None.

Associated background

None.

Differential diagnosis

Spindle cells such as the fibrocyte.

■ Spermatogenic cell

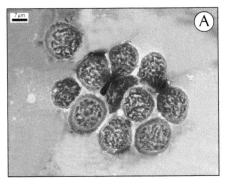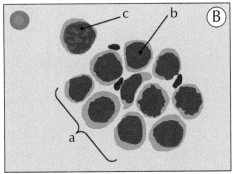

Figure 122 - Photomicrograph (A; Source: Courtesy of Carlo Masserdotti) and schematic representation (B) of the spermatogenic cell.

General characteristics and biological function

Cells of the germline, maturation of which leads to the spermatozoon.

Shape and size

Discrete cells (a), from medium to large in size, round in shape, with a high nuclear: cytoplasmic ratio.

Nucleus

Round, occupying most of the cell (b), consisting of lacy to coarse chromatin, often organized in large cords (c). Mitoses are frequent.

Cytoplasm

Scant, basophilic, with no particular detectable structures.

Location

Male genitalia, testis.

Cytoarchitectures

None.

Associated background

Often spermatozoa are found in the background.

Differential diagnosis

Immature lymphoid cells, erythroblast.

■ Spermatozoon

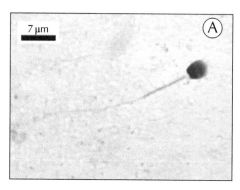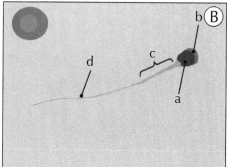

Figure 123 - Micrograph (A) and schematic representation (B) of the spermatozoon.

General characteristics and biological function

Mature cell responsible for oocyte fertilization during reproduction, arising from the spermatogenic cell division processes.

Shape and size

Spindle-shaped, filiform cells.

Nucleus

Small, with compact chromatin (a), characterized by a more clear apical area (b), the 'acrosome'.

Cytoplasm

Very scant, weakly basophilic, characterized by a proximal thickened area (c) and by a long flagellum (d).

Location

Male genitalia, mature testis, epididymis.

Cytoarchitectures

None. It can be found in association with Sertoli or epididymal cells.

Associated background

None.

Differential diagnosis

None.

■ Splenic macrophage

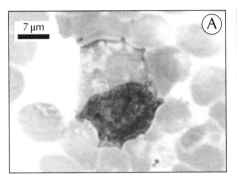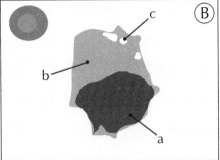

Figure 124 - Micrograph (A) and schematic representation (B) of the splenic macrophage.

General characteristics and biological function

This is a macrophage of the reticuloendothelial system of the spleen, mainly involved in catabolism of erythrocytes.

Shape and size

Comparable to that of a macrophage, pleomorphic, with low to intermediate nuclear:cytoplasmic ratio.

Nucleus

See Macrophage (a).

Cytoplasm

Large, grey (b), containing occasional optically empty vacuoles (c).

Location

Spleen.

Cytoarchitectures

None.

Associated background

Blood background.

Differential diagnosis

It is indistinguishable from other types of macrophages. In the spleen it can be confused with large lymphoid blasts (e.g. centroblast, immunoblast) of hyperplastic lymphoid white pulp.

■ Synoviocyte

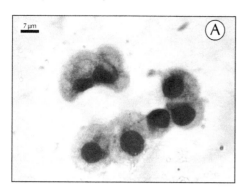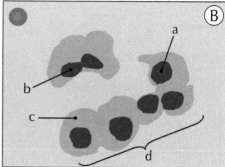

Figure 125 - Micrograph (A) and schematic representation (B) of the synoviocyte.

General characteristics and biological function

Cell which forms the lining of the synovial cavity.

Shape and size

Intermediate size, pleomorphic ranging from spindloid to epithelioid.

Nucleus

Round (a) to elongated–spindloid (b), with finely granular chromatin.

Cytoplasm

Moderately basophilic and finely granular (c).

Location

Joints, synovial cavity.

Cytoarchitectures

Small pavement cytoarchitectures (d).

Associated background

Proteinaceous, finely granular.

Differential diagnosis

Mesothelial cell.

Thymic epithelial cell

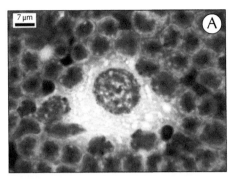
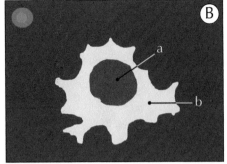

Figure 126 - Photomicrograph (A) and schematic representation (B) of the thymic epithelial cell.

General characteristics and biological function

Epithelial cell located in the thymus, involved in the maturation of T lymphocytes.

Shape and size

Very large cell, pleomorphic in shape.

Nucleus

Central, large, characterized by lacy to coarse chromatin (a).

Cytoplasm

Abundant and clear, with no particularly evident structures (b).

Location

Thymus.

Cytoarchitectures

Often detected in close connection with the small lymphocytes of the thymus.

Associated background

None.

Differential diagnosis

None.

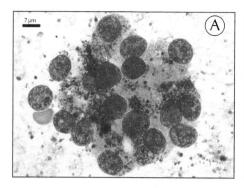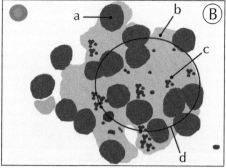

Figure 127 - Micrograph (A; Source: Courtesy of Carlo Masserdotti) and schematic representation (B) of the thyroid follicular cell.

General characteristics and biological function

Epithelial cell of the thyroid gland, responsible for thyroid hormone secretion.

Shape and size

Cuboidal, medium-sized, with low nuclear:cytoplasmic ratio.

Nucleus

Round, with finely stippled chromatin (a) and variably evident scattered nucleoli. Nuclei are homogeneous in this cytotype.

Cytoplasm

Large, bluish grey (b), in some cases containing dark blue pigments (c), interpreted as tyrosine accumulations.

Location

Thyroid.

Cytoarchitectures

These exfoliate cells in acinar (d) or 'honeycomb' cytoarchitectures, but can also exfoliate as isolated cells and in some cases as naked nuclei.

Associated background

Granules from the cytoplasm of the cells can be found as background.

Differential diagnosis

None.

■ Thyroid parafollicular cell

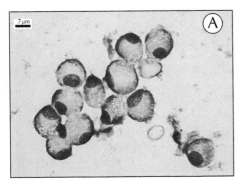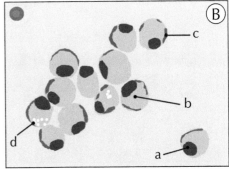

Figure 128 - Micrograph (A; Source: Courtesy of Carlo Masserdotti) and schematic representation (B) of the thyroid parafollicular cell.

General characteristics and biological function

Cell scattered in between thyroid follicles, responsible for the the production of calcitonin.

Shape and size

Large, round to ovoid cell, discrete, with low nuclear:cytoplasmic ratio.

Nucleus

The nucleus is round or ovoid, placed at the periphery of the cell (a), with reticular chromatin.

Cytoplasm

Abundant, grey (b), with occasional presence of more eosinophilic areas (c) and occasional cytoplasmic vacuolation (d).

Location

Thyroid.

Cytoarchitectures

None.

Associated background

None.

Differential diagnosis

Macrophages.

■ Tingible body macrophage

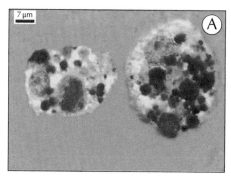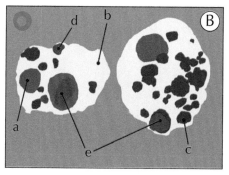

Figure 129 - Photomicrograph (A) and schematic representation (B) of the tingible body macrophage.

General characteristics and biological function

Resident macrophage of the lymph node and tissue-associated lymphatic nodules, responsible for phagocytosis of clones of lymphocytes triggered for elimination during clonal expansion.

Shape and size

See Macrophage.

Nucleus

See Macrophage (a).

Cytoplasm

See Macrophage (b). Typically contains fragments of basophilic cytoplasm (c) and nuclei (d) from the phagocytosed lymphocytes. Intact lymphocytes (e) are also detectable.

Location

Lymph node, tissue-associated lymphatic nodules: actively dividing follicle.

Cytoarchitectures

None.

Associated background

None.

Differential diagnosis

Other macrophages containing different pigments (haemosiderophage, melanophage, ceroid-laden macrophage).

■ Urothelial cell

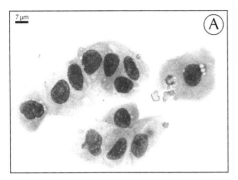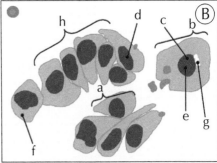

Figure 130 - Micrograph (A) and schematic representation (B) of the urothelial cell.

General characteristics and biological function

Epithelial cell lining the urinary bladder mucosa.

Shape and size

Small to large cell, with variable morphology. The typical morphology of these cells is pear-shaped (a), but cellular elements with polygonal (b) or spindloid morphology are detected. The degree of physiological anisocytosis of these cells is high.

Nucleus

Ovoid (c) to more elongated (d). The chromatin appears finely stippled, with visible nucleoli (e). Anisokaryosis can be evident physiologically.

Cytoplasm

Abundant, moderately basophilic (f), with occasional optically empty vacuoles (g).

Location

Bladder.

Cytoarchitectures

Isolated, palisade (h) or small pavement.

Associated background

None.

Differential diagnosis

Due to physiological anisocytosis and anisokaryosis they can resemble neoplastic cells.

Cytoarchitectures

■ Introduction

Cells that appear artificially scattered on a slide (in cytological preparations) derive from tissues in which such cells establish clearly defined mutual relations. The term cytoarchitecture refers to a group of cells maintaining a mutual organization that is similar to that they take in the organ from which they are derived.

Specific cytoarchitectures

Specific cytoarchitectures are those formed by groups of cells that retain their architecture, so as to appear as a whole structure, which can be directly compared with the structure present in histology. Among such specific cytoarchitectures are kidney glomeruli, which can keep their morphology unaltered in renal aspirates (Figure 131).

Generic cytoarchitectures

Generic cytoarchitectures are groups of cells which maintain their relationships intact, thus being a part of the structure that they form in their anatomical site of origin. Different cytotypes tend to form different cytoarchitectures. Epithelial cells form the greatest number of cytoarchitectures, while mesenchymal cells form many fewer. Discrete cells, by definition, do not form cytoarchitectures, except in very rare cases (e.g. *epithelioid macrophage*).

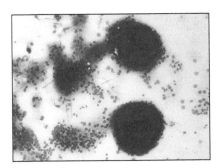

Figure 131 - Glomerular cytoarchitecture: kidney glomeruli may be preserved in their structure on the cytology sample.

Normal Cell Morphology in Canine and Feline Cytology: An Identification Guide,
First Edition. Written and translated by Lorenzo Ressel.
© 2018 John Wiley & Sons Ltd. Published 2018 by John Wiley & Sons Ltd.

■ Absence of cytoarchitecture (or sheets of cells)

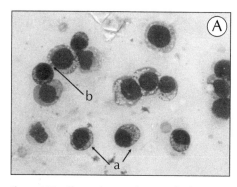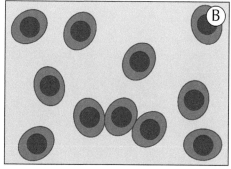

Figure 132 - Photomicrograph (A) and schematic representation (B) of absence of cytoarchitecture.

Morphological characteristics

Cells that do not establish any mutual connection, either directly or by interposition of matrix, exfoliate on the preparation just like single cells (discrete) (a). This type of distribution, which does not form a cytoarchitecture, is sometimes called 'sheets of cells'.

Although cells are individual, in some areas of the slide, due to a high concentration, 'mechanical' aggregates of cells may appear (b). For the purpose of distinguishing such cells from true cytoarchitectures, it is advisable to observe the margins of the cellular elements in contact, which, in this case, are noticeably sharper than those observed in the case of clusters of epithelial cells.

Cellular lineage

Round cells and mesenchymal cells. Cells that are not resident in the tissues. Exuded inflammatory cells.

Examples of typical cytotypes

Small lymphocyte and other lymphoid cells, mast cell, macrophage, bone marrow cells, osteoblast.

■ Acinar cytoarchitecture

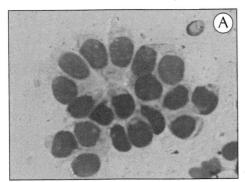 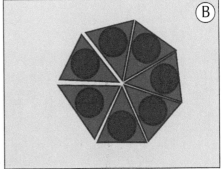

Figure 133 - Photomicrograph (A) and schematic representation (B) of acinar cytoarchitecture.

Morphological characteristics

In acinar cytoarchitectures, cells are arranged in a circle to form a structure resembling a glandular acinus, at the centre of which it may be possible to identify a lumen. These structures are indicative of exfoliated cells' tendency to maintain the morphology of glands from the tissue of origin.

Cellular lineage

Epithelial; typical of glandular epithelia.

Examples of typical cytotypes

Anal sac apocrine cell, apocrine cell.

■ Honeycomb cytoarchitecture

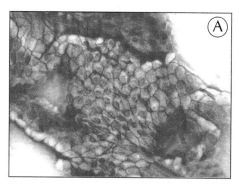 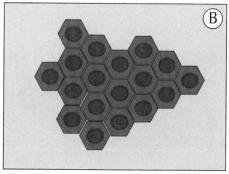

Figure 134 - Micrograph (A; Source: Courtesy of Carlo Masserdotti) and schematic representation (B) of honeycomb cytoarchitecture.

Morphological characteristics

'Honeycomb' cytoarchitecture is similar to squamous cytoarchitecture, however, it is formed by cubic and regular elements that resemble the hexagonal cells of beehives. The cells that constitute this cytoarchitecture tend not to create multiple layers.

Cellular lineage

Epithelial.

Examples of typical cytotypes

Prostate cell, gastric superficial mucous cell, thyroid follicular cell.

■ Palisade cytoarchitectures

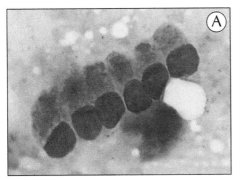 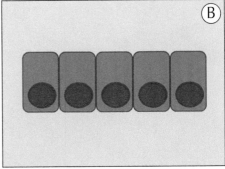

Figure 135 - Micrograph (A) and schematic representation (B) of palisade cytoarchitecture.

Morphological characteristics

In palisade cytoarchitectures, cells are arranged one beside the other, organized to form a row of elements that resembles a palisade. This cytoarchitecture can be composed of cells either of the same or different type (e.g. *ciliated epithelial cell+goblet cell* in the respiratory tract).

Cellular lineage

Epithelial cells; often columnar epithelia such as the one in the respiratory tract.

Examples of typical cytotypes

Gastric mucous surface cell, ciliated epithelial cell, biliary cell, Sertoli cell, epididymal cell, enterocyte.

■ Papillary cytoarchitecture

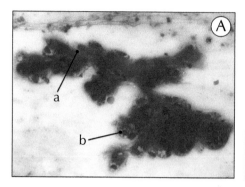 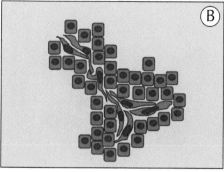

Figure 136 - Photomicrograph (A) and schematic representation (B) of papillary cytoarchitecture.

Morphological characteristics

This type of cytoarchitecture is more typical of anatomical structures that occur in pathological conditions. It was included in this section for the sake of completeness. Cells that form a papillary cytoarchitecture are of two types: supporting stromal cells (a) and external epithelial cells (b).

Cellular lineage

Mesenchymal and epithelial forming papillae, which are often associated with hyperplastic phenomena.

Examples of typical cytotypes

Mammary cell, myoepithelial cell, mammary foam cell, fibroblast.

■ Pavement cytoarchitecture

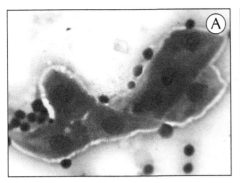 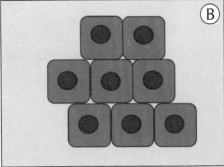

Figure 137 - Photomicrograph (A) and schematic representation (B) of pavement cytoarchitecture.

Morphological characteristics

Pavement cytoarchitectures appear as a group of cells arranged in a way that reminds one of a tiled floor. Cellular margins do not overlap and cells appear neatly arranged on the same plane.

Cellular lineage

Epithelial; in particular lining epithelia (e.g. mesothelium or epidermis).

Examples of typical cytotypes

Squamous epithelial cell, conjunctival squamous cell, mesothelial cell.

■ Perivascular cytoarchitecture

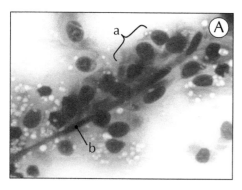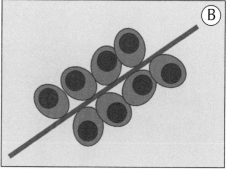

Figure 138 - Photomicrograph (A; Source: Courtesy of Carlo Masserdotti) and schematic representation (B) of perivascular cytoarchitecture.

Morphological characteristics

Cells that form a perivascular cytoarchitecture (a) surround recognizable capillaries (b).

Cellular lineage

Mesenchymal and epithelial.

Examples of typical cytotypes

Leydig cell, hepatocyte, endocrine cells.

■ Solid three-dimensional cytoarchitecture

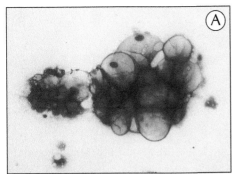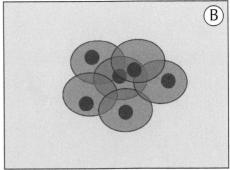

Figure 139 - Photomicrograph (A) and schematic representation (B) of solid three-dimensional cytoarchitecture.

Morphological characteristics

In solid three-dimensional cytoarchitectures, cells are arranged to form structures that are not on the same level; they consist of multiple layers of interconnected cells.

Cellular lineage

Mesenchymal and epithelial.

Examples of typical cytotypes

Adipocyte, sebocyte.

■ Storiform cytoarchitecture

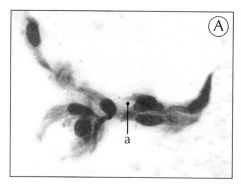
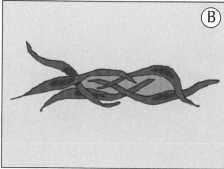

Figure 140 - Photomicrograph (A) and schematic representation (B) of storiform cytoarchitecture.

Morphological characteristics

Storiform cytoarchitectures consist of a weave of spindle-shaped cells, together with variable amounts of interspersed matrix (a).

Cellular lineage

Mesenchymal.

Examples of typical cytotypes

Fibroblast, fibrocyte.

■ Trabecular cytoarchitectures

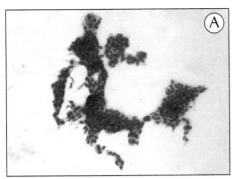 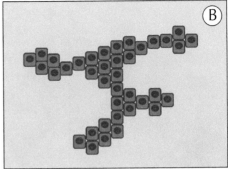

Figure 141 - Photomicrograph (A) and schematic representation (B) of trabecular cytoarchitecture.

Morphological characteristics

Trabecular cytoarchitectures feature large cellular aggregates with a branching pattern.

Cellular lineage

Epithelial cells.

Examples of typical cytotypes

Hepatocyte, hepatoid cell, mammary gland cell.

■ Tubular cytoarchitecture

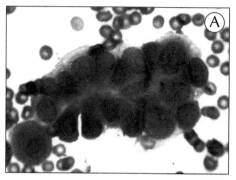 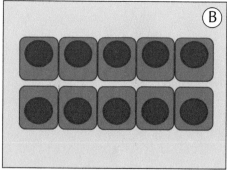

Figure 142 - Photomicrograph (A) and schematic representation (B) of tubular cytoarchitecture.

Morphological characteristics

Cells that form tubular cytoarchitectures are arranged on two opposing rows that resemble a palisade. A lumen can be seen in between the two rows.

Cellular lineage

Epithelial (often glandular) cells.

Examples of typical cytotypes

Renal tubular cell, apocrine cell.

Background

◼ Introduction

The background is the material found in conjunction with the sampled cells from a certain area, with which it is associated in the composition of the specimen. It often indicates the presence of some organic non-cellular matrix. Nonetheless, it is commonly accepted that the background represented by blood contamination, which contains cellular elements (*erythrocytes* and *leucocytes*), can also be considered a 'background'. It may be absent or present. When present, it may be composed of blood or non-cellular matrix. Often, various types of background and matrices merge together to form a complex background.

◼ Absence of background

When no matrix interposed between cells nor significant amount of contamination blood can be found on the sample, the background is considered to be absent (Figure 143).

◼ Blood background

Blood background can be found in the majority of cytological preparations. It is composed of blood (blood contamination), which comes from vessels that are damaged during the sampling process (Figure 144). The presence of this type of background is frequent and often non-specific. It may simply be caused by the operator's sampling procedures, or be due to a large quantity of blood in the target organ (e.g. the spleen).

The presence of *platelets* (which must be detected within the background – Figure 144a) is an important feature of blood contamination for the purpose of distinguishing it from real blood collections (e.g. haematomas). *Erythrocytes* can aggregate in some areas and lose their characteristic morphology (Figure 144b).

Normal Cell Morphology in Canine and Feline Cytology: An Identification Guide,
First Edition. Written and translated by Lorenzo Ressel.
© 2018 John Wiley & Sons Ltd. Published 2018 by John Wiley & Sons Ltd.

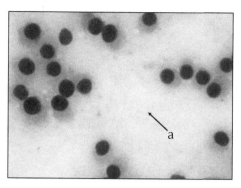

Figure 143 - No background: in areas that are interposed between cells (a), there is no consistent structure or material worthy of note.

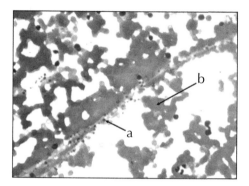

Figure 144 - Blood background: presence of red erythrocytes and platelets (a); erythrocytes in some areas agglomerate (b).

■ Background composed of matrix

Background composed of matrix can be detected either in focal areas or throughout the slide. The matrix background can be characteristic of certain types of tissue and cell types, or, in some cases, it may be shared between different tissues. The matrix may be generic or specific.

Generic matrices

Generic matrices are substances whose category is definable only on a broad basis while their specific nature is not. These are fatty, proteinaceous and mixed matrices.

Fatty matrix

Fatty matrix is composed of lipid globules (micelles), which can either be widespread or localized in some areas of the preparation (Figure 145a). Such globules may vary in size and appear clear and unstained to the eye. This matrix often derives from tissues with high fat component from which (during sample preparation) the lipids spread onto the background of the preparation. This type of matrix is also present in areas characterized by vigorous production of fat-rich substances (e.g. sebum).

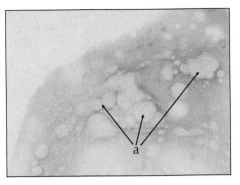

Figure 145 - Fat background: the presence of considerable amounts of optically empty lipid micelles (a) is characteristic of this type of background.

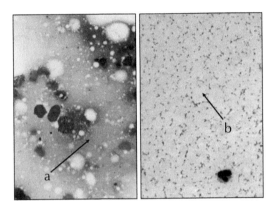

Figure 146 - Proteinaceous background: the presence of pink amorphous material is evident in the sample. The proteinaceous matrix may present as amorphous/'liquid' (a), or finely granular (b).

Proteinaceous matrix

Proteinaceous matrix is usually well distributed in the whole preparation. It is characterized by the presence of an amorphous to granular substance. It may appear pink (eosinophilic), compact (Figure 146a) or varyingly corpuscular (Figure 146b). This non-specific matrix can have various origins from different proteins. It is often present in contexts where there is secretion (e.g. apocrine gland), or may characterize the protein component of inflammatory exudation (oedema).

Mixed fat–proteinaceous matrix

The fat–proteinaceous matrix is an example of a complex matrix. This type of matrix features areas consisting typically of proteinaceous matrix (Figure 147) as well as areas containing lipid micelles (Figure 145). This type of matrix is typical of the lactating mammary gland.

Specific matrices

These are special matrices whose morphology can be used to perform a more precise classification of the substance of origin.

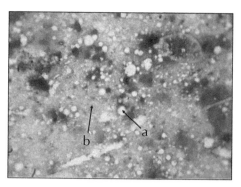

Figure 147 - Fat–proteinaceous background: example of simultaneous presence of fat matrix (a) and proteinaceous matrix (b) to form a complex background.

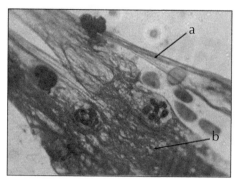

Figure 148 - Mucinous matrix: thin filaments of pink material (a) organized into a loose reticular pattern (b) which entraps the cells.

Mucinous matrix

Mucinous matrix (mucus) is usually localized multifocally within the slide and it features long pinkish filaments (Figure 148a), which can be intertwined (Figure 148b), often forming nets that trap various cells. This matrix appears stringy but not properly fibrillar. Its margins are well delimited from the areas without background.

Collagenous matrix

Collagenous matrix is composed entirely of collagen. It usually has a multifocal distribution and is often associated with cells of fibroblastic nature (fibroblasts and fibrocytes). It appears pinkish and clearly fibrillar (Figure 149).

Osteoid matrix

Osteoid is bone matrix that has not yet mineralized. Ninety percent of the osteoid matrix is composed of collagen, while the remaining 10% features mostly proteoglycans. It appears as a fairly homogeneous matrix (Figure 150), with some darker/basophilic and denser areas (a), which suggest early mineralization. Some areas may feature a more pronounced fibrillar-like structure (b), however, they are not comparable to those of collagenous matrix. This matrix is often characterized by a focal distribution and the presence of *osteoblasts* and *osteoclasts*.

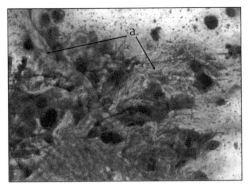

Figure 149 - Collagenous matrix: predominant presence of pink material that forms clear fibrils, which are variable in size (a).

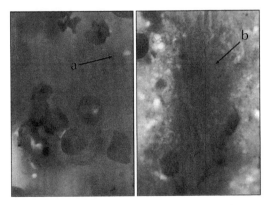

Figure 150 - Osteoid matrix: pinkish matrix that, in some areas, is amorphous, with intensification in the colour in some areas (a). In other areas it may tend to form semi-fibrillar structures (b).

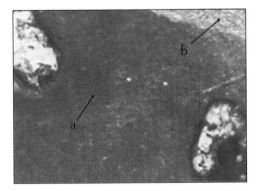

Figure 151 - Chondroid matrix: the presence of large areas occupied by diffuse, homogeneous amorphous substance, pink in colour (a), which in some areas may tend to form fine granules (b).

Chondroid matrix

The chondroid matrix is composed of 40% collagen and 60% proteoglycans. It appears as a widespread (in the entire preparation, sometimes described as 'lakes'), purple, homogeneous, more watery and non-fibrillar matrix (Figure 151a). In some areas, it may be finely granular (Figure 151b). *Chondroblasts* are associated with this matrix.

Morphological alterations of cells

■ Introduction

Morphological alterations are special modifications affecting the physiology and morphology of a given cytotype. They indicate some kind of pathological process. The purpose of this book is not to deal with the morphological characteristics of each pathological entity (e.g. morphology of carcinoma vs. sarcoma cells), but to give an overview of the individual changes. Morphological alterations of cells fall into three broad categories of pathological processes: degenerative alterations, alterations related to cellular death, and progressive–dysplastic alterations. In cytology, the latter are referred as 'atypical features', or, if referring to a malignant neoplasm, 'criteria of malignancy'.

■ Morphological alterations related to cellular degeneration

Morphological alterations related to cellular degeneration usually occur because of abnormal accumulation of substances within the cytoplasm (Figure 152a). Intracellular accumulations (for example, steatosis in the *hepatocyte*) must be considered pathological in cells that do not normally contain material in the cytoplasm in large amounts (e.g. *adipocyte* or *sebocyte*). The presence of these inclusions is a symptom of cellular distress linked to the impossibility of performing normal turnover of the specific substance. These cells may eventually die or revert to normal.

■ Morphological alterations linked to cellular death

In cytological terms, alterations linked to cellular death can be observed mainly within the nucleus. They are classified as karyorrhexis/karyolysis and karyopyknosis.

Normal Cell Morphology in Canine and Feline Cytology: An Identification Guide,
First Edition. Written and translated by Lorenzo Ressel.
© 2018 John Wiley & Sons Ltd. Published 2018 by John Wiley & Sons Ltd.

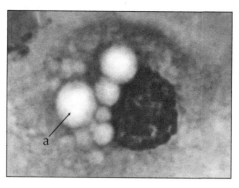

Figure 152 - Cell degeneration: presence of vacuolation (a) that indents the nucleus, in a cytotype which does not present with intracytoplasmic vacuoles in physiological conditions.

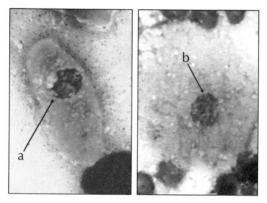

Figure 153 - Karyorrhexis/karyolysis: the nuclear morphology is altered, with vesicular and fragmented areas (a), leading to nuclear dissolution (b).

Karyorrhexis/karyolysis

In karyorrhexis, the nucleus loses its characteristic round shape, and the chromatin appears, irregular in shape in some areas (Figure 153a). It is fragmented into small, separated parts (Figure 153b), and, in the case of karyolysis, it can even disappear. At times, this morphological alteration may lead the observer into considering it a mitotic figure, thus it is important to pay particular attention to this aspect.

Karyopyknosis (or pyknosis)

In karyopyknosis, the nucleus is 'hypercondensed', compact and very dark, so as not to show any difference in the context of the two chromatin types (hetero- and eu-). In cells with a round nucleus, the nucleus decreases in diameter and keeps the same shape (Figure 154a). In cells with a polylobed nucleus, fragmentation and condensation of single parts is possible (Figure 154b).

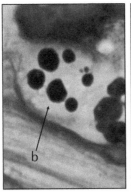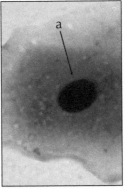

Figure 154 - Karyopyknosis: the nuclei of cells are small, condensed and dark (a). In the case of a lobulated nucleus, fragmentation can occur (b) during the process of karyopyknosis.

■ Atypical features

'Atypical feature' refers to a morphological feature, neither degenerative nor linked to cellular death, that is associated with a typical morphology and that clearly distinguishes it from the normal cytotype. These features may be indicative of dysplastic alterations, due to concomitant inflammatory insult, but also progressive hyperplastic or neoplastic changes. Except for rare atypical features, which almost always indicate neoplastic cellular characteristics, generally speaking, one cannot use a single atypical feature alone to distinguish between dysplasia or neoplasia. Hyperplastic, dysplastic cells or benign neoplastic cells can have overlapping atypical features. In neoplasia, observing more than one atypical feature (classically more than three) in the majority of the cells of the same cytotype is suggestive of malignant neoplastic transformation, hence the the term 'criteria of malignancy'.

It should also be noted that atypical features must be compared and interpreted considering the normal cytotype morphology. In this regard, two general rules seem appropriate.

- Some cytotypes normally exhibit a degree of atypical features (e.g. *urothelial cell* – anisocytosis; *immunoblast* – high number of mitotic figures). Those should be evaluated in this context with due caution.
- There are special cases of cancer that do not show morphological signs of their malignancy through the usual atypical features, but which are indeed tumours and behave aggressively.

As this does not represent the main focus of this book, for a thorough characterization of atypical features in the context of individual cytotypes (e.g. tumours arising from a particular cell type), please refer to current diagnostic cytology textbooks. This chapter will deal separately with the morphological changes that determine the appearance of atypical features. Atypical features are divided into cellular, cytoplasmic and nuclear.

Atypical cellular features

Atypical cellular features are those that affect the whole cell. These include hyper-cellularity, bi- to multinucleation, cellular pleomorphism, anisocytosis, appearance of a cytotype in a non-typical area, nuclear–cytoplasmic maturation asynchrony and increased nuclear:cytoplasmic ratio.

Hypercellularity

Hypercellularity is a criterion that simply indicates a high number of cells of a particular cytotype in the sample. This occurrence can depend on several factors.

- The type of sampling (more or less aggressive) can result in the production of a preparation that is variable in cellularity, even if it comes from the same site (e.g. scraping vs. imprint).
- The cellularity of a cytotype in a sample may depend on its greater readiness to exfoliate compared to other cytotypes. In this respect, it must be considered that discrete cells, because of their natural condition of not being in contact with other cells, are easily aspirated. On the contrary, mesenchymal cells, embedded in extracellular matrix, tend not to have such a feature.
- The cellularity of a sample depends on the actual number of cells of the cytotype in question present within the area (e.g. in a neoplastic proliferation more cells are expected compared to the normal tissue of origin).
- De-differentiation processes, which can occur in some pathological phenomena such as neoplastic transformation, favour the loss of a cell's normal ability to remain attached to another one (directly in the case of epithelial cells, indirectly in the case of mesenchymal cells).

It must be noted that that only the last two factors, among the causes taken into consideration in this analysis, represent a true expression of 'atypia'. A cautious evaluation of this parameter is therefore strongly suggested, especially if it is to be used as part of a diagnostic process.

Bi- to multinucleation

The presence of more than one nucleus in a cell that normally hosts only one usually indicates improper cellular division and failed cytokinesis. Exceptions are the cyto-types that can form multinucleated cells (syncitia) as a normal behaviour (e.g. macrophage). Multinucleated cells contain from three to several nuclei within a single cytoplasm (Figure 155a), even if belonging to cell types that normally host only one nucleus. Often, if this change represents an atypical feature, the cell nuclei display some degree of anisokaryosis among them (see Anisokaryosis). This factor is useful to differentiate these cells from normal multinucleated cytotypes (e.g. osteoclast).

The presence of binucleate cells can be, in some cases, characteristic of certain types of neoplastic processes, resulting in the appearance of 'insect head' cells (Figure 155b). Imperfect cytokinesis may rarely determine a third atypical form of multinucleation called 'micronucleus' (Figure 155c), in which a small nucleus appears next to the normal one.

Cellular pleomorphism

Sometimes, alterations of the cellular shape within the same cytotype may be observed. Although some authors often consider this feature as part of the 'anisocytosis'

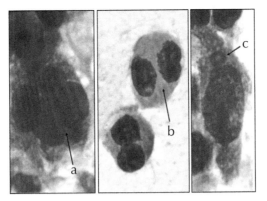

Figure 155 - Binucleation, multinucleation. In the cytoplasm of the cells depicted, four nuclei are observed (a). Two nuclei with typical 'insect head' morphology are evident (b). One normal nucleus accompanied by one 'micronucleus' is also evident (c).

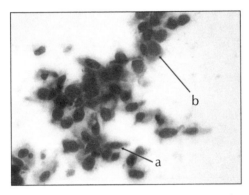

Figure 156 - Cellular pleomorphism: cells belonging to the same cytotype show spindle/fusiform (a) and round (b) shapes.

concept (see Anisocytosis), cytotypes that are normally very homogeneous can, during dysplastic or neoplastic changes, take on different shapes without necessarily undergoing substantial alterations in cell size (Figure 156).

Anisocytosis

Anisocytosis refers to the appearance of cells that, despite belonging to the same cytotype, show significant differences in cell size (Figure 157a). This alteration is normally associated with anisokaryosis.

The terms 'macrocytosis' (directly associated with 'macrokaryosis') or 'cellular gigantism' are used for exceptionally large cells, in the context of normally sized cells of a single cytotype (Figure 157b). The latter aspect appears regularly in malignant neoplastic transformation.

Presence of a cell type in atypical area (metastasis)

This is one of the very few atypical features which, individually, provides a strong indication of cellular neoplastic malignant transformation. Morphologically speaking, it is based on the recognition of a cytotype as not being part of the normal population (Figure 158), given the knowledge of normal cytotypes of a

161

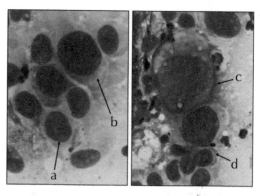

Figure 157 - Anisocytosis: cells belonging to the same cytotype show significantly different size (a vs. b); in some cases, the difference in the cell size (c vs. d) is so marked that justifies the use of the term 'macrokaryosis' or 'cell gigantism'.

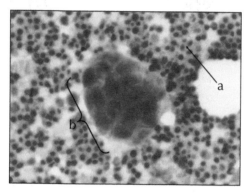

Figure 158 - Presence of a cell type in atypical area: in the context of a normal lymph node population (a), there are squamous cells, grouped in a cluster, indicative of metastatic epithelial cells (b).

given organ (see Chapter 2, Distribution of cells in tissues and organs). The presence of a cytotype that is completely incompatible with any of those residing in the area of the organ is a strong indication of a metastatic neoplastic process, particularly if detected in typical target organs of metastatic processes and associated with additional atypical features. However, it must be noted that in some rare cases and in specific areas, a phenomenon called 'metaplasia' can occur (see Atypical cytoplasmic features) which is not necessarily neoplastic. Metaplasia may determine the appearance of ectopic cytotypes (for example, the appearance of *chondroblasts* during chondroid metaplasia of the mammary gland stroma; appearance of *rubriblasts*, *rubricytes* or *megakaryocytes* in the spleen and liver in extramedullary erythropoiesis) as a consequence of chronic inflammation or other stimuli.

Nuclear–cytoplasmic maturation asynchrony

In some cytotypes, maturation of the cytoplasm (with the appearance of particular structures or shapes) occurs in conjunction with maturation of the nucleus which, usually, acquires characteristics that are attributable to a lower metabolic or replicative activity (reduction in size, increase in heterochromatin component). In these cytotypes, during the course of alterations induced by dysplastic or neoplastic

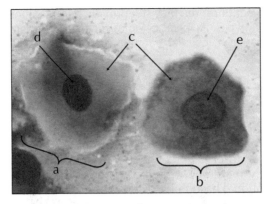

Figure 159 - Nuclear–cytoplasmic maturation asynchrony: comparison between a normal mature keratinocyte (a) and a neoplastic one (b). The shape of both presents as polygonal/angular (c), typical of a proper cytoplasmic maturation, while the nuclei differ. The normal keratinocyte exhibits condensed chromatin (d), while the neoplastic cell shows an immature morphology, with euchromatin and presence of a prominent nucleolus (e).

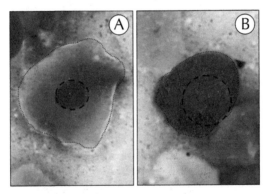

Figure 160 - Increase in nuclear:cytoplasmic ratio: normal mature keratinocyte (A) shows low ratio (dotted lines). The neoplastic keratinocyte (B) in comparison shows increased ratio (dotted lines).

phenomena (e.g. *keratinized squamous epithelial cell*), it is possible to observe a discrepancy in maturation between the nucleus and the cytoplasm (Figure 159). The cytoplasm may appear mature (typical of differentiated cytotypes), while the nucleus may still be immature (larger with more euchromatin and nucleoli).

Increase in nuclear:cytoplasmic ratio

An increase in nuclear:cytoplasmic ratio in a cell type that normally has a low or intermediate ratio is indicative of de-differentiation to a more immature form (Figure 160). This character of atypia is seen in both dysplastic and neoplastic phenomena.

Atypical cytoplasmic features

Atypical cytoplasmic features are alterations of cytoplasmic morphologies that are considered normal within a specific cytotype. Generally, atypical cytoplasmic features, when considered as criteria of malignancy in neoplasms, are weaker indicators compared with nuclear ones. Yet, they still provide important information about the differentiation of cytotypes. Atypical cytoplasmic features are hyperbasophilia, de-differentiation, metaplasia, cellular cannibalism (emperipolesis) and cytoplasmic microvacuolation.

Cytoplasmic hyperbasophilia

Cytoplasmic basophilia indicates high protein synthesis (see Chapter 1, Cellular biology and cytological interpretation: the philosophy behind the system). A given cytotype is usually characterized by a relatively well-defined cytoplasm colour. This may get closer to that of hyperbasophilia if the cytoplasm of the cell features abnormally increased protein synthesis (Figure 161). There are cases in which the exceptional basophilia of the cytoplasm renders the nucleus barely visible.

This feature is obviously to be assessed in the context of the knowledge of the normal cytoplasmic staining affinity of the cytotype, as some cell types may be physiologically hyperbasophilic (e.g. *immunoblast*).

De-differentiation (anaplasia)

The cytoplasm of some cytotypes is characterized by specific structures that indicate a certain cell differentiation (for example, *mast cell*: the presence of intracytoplasmic granules). In some cases, the differentiation process also results in a specific cell shape. The reduced presence or complete absence of such cytoplasmic structures (or morphology change) is part of a de-differentiation process, which is typical of neoplastic transformations (Figure 162).

Metaplasia

Metaplasia refers to the transformation of a cytotype into a different cell type, traditionally belonging to the same embryological derivation (Figure 163). Examples of metaplasia are *fibroblasts* that become *osteoblasts*, or *ciliated epithelial cells* that turn into *keratinized squamous epithelial cells*. This transformation often appears in conjunction with hyperplastic, inflammatory or neoplastic phenomena. It is important to distinguish this phenomenon from the metastatic process.

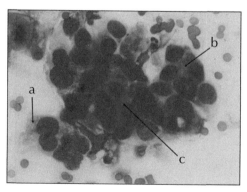

Figure 161 - Cytoplasmic hyperbasophilia: cells of the same cell type show progressive basophilia: from a moderately basophilic cytoplasm (a), to a basophilic cytoplasm (b), to an hyperbasophilic cytoplasm (c).

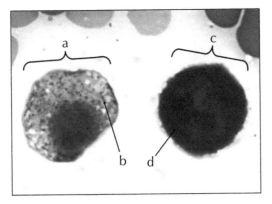

Figure 162 - De-differentiation (anaplasia): the neoplastic mast cell (a) shows rare intracytoplasmic granules (b), when compared with a healthy mast cell (c), whose cytoplasm is uniformly packed with granules (d).

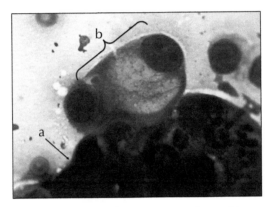

Figure 163 - Metaplasia: during proliferation of non-secretory cell types (a), some cells assume a 'signet-ring shape', which suggests transformation into a secretory cell type (b).

Cellular cannibalism (emperipolesis)

In some neoplastic transformations, cells which usually do not carry out phagocytosis can engulf (Figure 164) cells belonging to either other cytotypes (Figure 164a) or belonging to their same cytotype.

It is not always easy to ascertain, especially when inflammatory cells are phagocytosed, if cells are actually overlapping. In such cases, the appearance of a curvature in the intracytoplasmic structures, such as the nucleus, can be a helpful clue (Figure 164b) to support real cell engulfment. However, some authors suggest that this phenomenon is not a real phagocytosis but an extreme invagination of the cell membrane around another cell, which is known as 'emperipolesis'.

Cytoplasmic microvacuolation

The presence of microvacuolations, at times localized in specific areas such as the perinuclear area (Figure 165a), suggests altered metabolic activity. This may be found in cells affected by dysplastic and neoplastic phenomena.

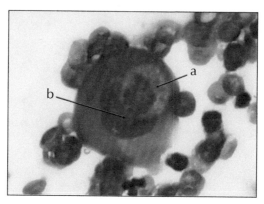

Figure 164 - Cannibalism/emperipolesis: an epithelial squamous cell (physiologically not phagocytosing) has engulfed another cell (a) which exhibits a mitotic figure. The internalization of the cell, rather than a simple overlap, is testified by the modification of the nuclear shape of the squamous cell (b).

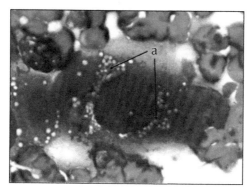

Figure 165 - Cytoplasmic microvacuolization: presence of very small, clear vacuoles, preferentially localized in the perinuclear area (a).

Atypical nuclear features

Atypical nuclear features are specific alterations of the nucleus and subnuclear components of the cell. These characters are extremely important elements in the assessment of neoplastic cell's malignancy and include: anisokaryosis, nuclear pleomorphism, convolutions and indentation of the nucleus, altered chromatin patterns, nuclear moulding, atypical mitoses, increased numbers of mitotic figures, prominent nucleolus, multiple nucleoli, anisonucleoliosis, teratonucleoliosis (atypical nucleolar morphology), macronucleoliosis and margination of nucleoli.

Anisokaryosis

Anisokaryosis refers to a tendency of some cell nuclei to be significantly different in size despite belonging to the same cytotype (Figure 166). Currently, there is no universal size variation threshold determining when an alteration in size is to be considered anisokaryosis. This criterion is typical of cells affected by neoplastic transformation. It is worth noting, however, that different cytotypes display different degrees of physiological anisokaryosis, therefore, anisokaryosis must be evaluated in conjunction with the cytotype being considered (e.g. *urothelial cells* are physiologically anisokaryotic).

Nuclear pleomorphism

Nuclear pleomorphism refers to a change in the shape of the nucleus, within the same cytotype (Figure 167). Again, it is appropriate to start with analysis of the cytotype's morphology and its typical physiological variation range. This feature is usually inextricably linked to cellular pleomorphism.

Convolutions and nuclear indentations

The nuclear membrane can undergo morphological alterations resulting in the appearance of indentations (folds inside the core of the nuclear membrane) or nuclear convolutions (areas of the nucleus that feature lobes folding back on themselves) (Figure 168). In order to be classified as atypical features, these changes must appear in cytotypes that do not normally have such physiological characteristics.

Altered chromatin patterns

The morphology of the chromatin usually differs depending on the cytotype. Altered chromatin pattern often refers to the appearance of a more immature chromatin morphology, compared to that typical of the normal cell (Figure 169).

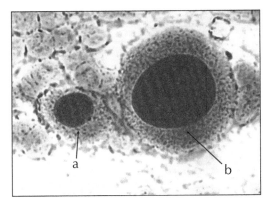

Figure 166 - Anisokaryosis: cells belonging to the same cell type show different sizes of nucleus (a vs. b). In this case cells are also exhibiting anisocytosis.

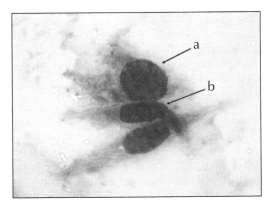

Figure 167 - Nuclear pleomorphism: cells belonging to the same cell type show different nuclear shapes, either round (a) or fusiform (b).

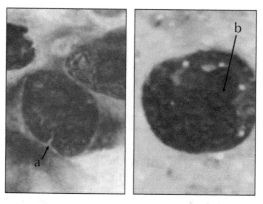

Figure 168 - Nuclear convolutions and indentations: the nuclear membrane is characterized by indentations (a) and convolutions (b).

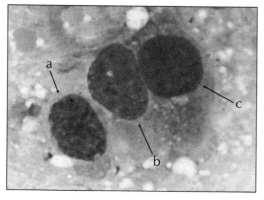

Figure 169 - Altered chromatin patterns: in the context of the same cell type different chromatin patterns are detected – coarse (a), finely stippled (b), clumped (c).

Nuclear moulding

Nuclear moulding is an alteration in which two or more nuclei belonging to contiguous cells (or to the same multinucleated cell) are crushed against each other so as to alter the nuclear morphology and, in some cases, result in an apparent fusion (Figure 170). It is appropriate to differentiate this atypical feature from cellular overlap, a common phenomenon occurring in cytological preparations. In the latter case, mutual morphological alterations of the nuclei are less likely to take place.

Atypical mitoses

Atypical mitosis refers to a mitotic figure that deviates from the typical morphology of traditional mitosis (see Chapter 1, Cellular biology and cytological interpretation: the philosophy behind the system). In order to identify this alteration, it is useful observe an asymmetrical distribution of the chromatin material compared to an imaginary symmetrical axis. Atypical mitoses also exhibit chromatin bodies that are detached from the two main segregation areas (Figure 171).

168

An increase in the number of mitotic figures is a decisive parameter in the assessment of cell proliferation. It denotes a high replicative activity of the cells. This parameter must be calibrated considering the normal mitotic activity of the cytotype. Certain cell types normally feature a high mitotic activity (e.g. *basal cell*), while in other cells, the presence of a single mitotic figure may already be indicative of atypia and in some cases malignancy (e.g. *chondroblast*).

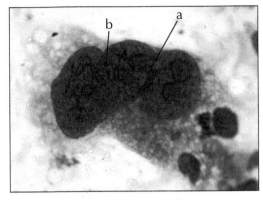

Figure 170 - Nuclear moulding: the nuclei of the trinucleated cell in the figure are in close contact, with modification of membrane outline (a), or apparent fusion (b).

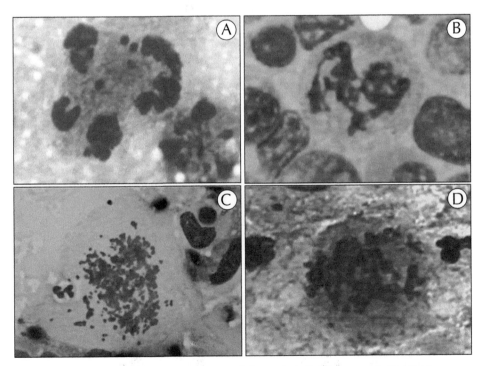

Figure 171 - Atypical mitotic figures: segregation of chromatin material asymmetrically (A), bizarre figures (B), irregular 'explosion-like' distribution of chromatin fragments (C, D).

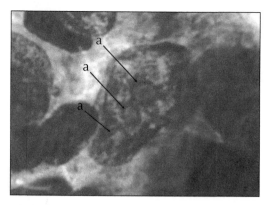

Figure 172 - Multiple nucleoli: three nucleoli (a) are observed in a cytotype where one is the norm.

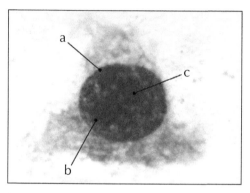

Figure 173 - Anisonucleoliosis: nucleoli vary in size from small (a), to medium (b), to large (c).

Prominent nucleolus

In cytotypes characterized by a non-visible nucleolus in physiological conditions, the nucleolus can become visible and it is considered indicative of increased metabolic status. It must be noted that many cytotypes feature prominent nucleoli under physiological conditions due to their high basal metabolic activity. In the nucleus of the neoplastic cell represented in Figure 159, the presence of a nucleolus in the neoplastic cells (b), which does not appear in a healthy counterpart (a), is quite obvious.

Multiple nucleoli

In physiological conditions, most mature cells, despite being metabolically very active, do not feature numerous nucleoli. As an exception, extremely immature cells can feature numerous nucleoli under normal physiological conditions (e.g. *rubriblast*). In neoplastic cell transformation, the number of nucleoli can increase substantially (Figure 172).

Anisonucleoliosis

Anisonucleoliosis refers to different sizes of nucleoli within the same cell nucleus or compared between cells of the same cytotype (Figure 173). This feature is often detected in neoplastic transformation.

Teratonucleoliosis refers to morphological alteration of the nucleolus, which results in the loss of the typical round shape. A cell affected by this alteration may feature a nucleus with a rather unusually shaped nucleolus: triangular, spindle-like, elongated or kidney-shaped (Figure 174).

Macronucleoliosis

The increased size of the nucleolus represents an important morphological alteration. Macronucleoliosis refers to a nucleolus with a considerably increased size (Figure 175). A nucleolus that is larger than an *erythrocyte* is a strong indication of a cell's malignant neoplastic transformation (criteria of malignancy).

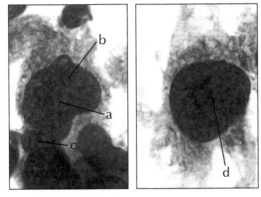

Figure 174 - Teratonucleoliosis (atypical nucleoli): nucleoli are characterized by bizarre-elongated (a), triangular (b), cuboidal (c), bilobed (d) shapes.

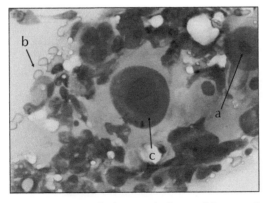

Figure 175 - Macronucleoliosis: presence of a large nucleolus (a) of the same size of an erythrocyte (b); sometimes, it is possible to identify larger (giant) nucleoli (c).

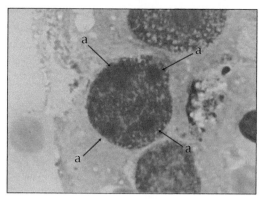

Figure 176 - Margination of nucleoli: nucleoli are arranged at the periphery of the nucleus, in close contact with the nuclear membrane (a).

Margination of nucleoli

The margination of nucleoli is an alteration in which the nucleoli are found in close contact with the nuclear membrane (Figure 176). It should be noted that this feature is also typical of some cytotypes (e.g. *centroblast*).

Visual index

The purpose of this section is to provide a quick summary of the morphological features, size and mutual maturative relationship of different cell cytotypes.

Four figures represent all the different cytotypes via schematic representation (diagram). The diagram of each cell is in scale with respect to the other cytotypes and in scale to the red blood cell reference diagram on the top right. Close to each cell diagram is the name of the cytotype, so the reader can refer to its detailed description in Chapter 3, Cytotypes.

Grey arrows between cell types represent a maturative relationship (e.g. the *macrophage* originates from differentiation of the *monocyte*).

Normal Cell Morphology in Canine and Feline Cytology: An Identification Guide,
First Edition. Written and translated by Lorenzo Ressel.

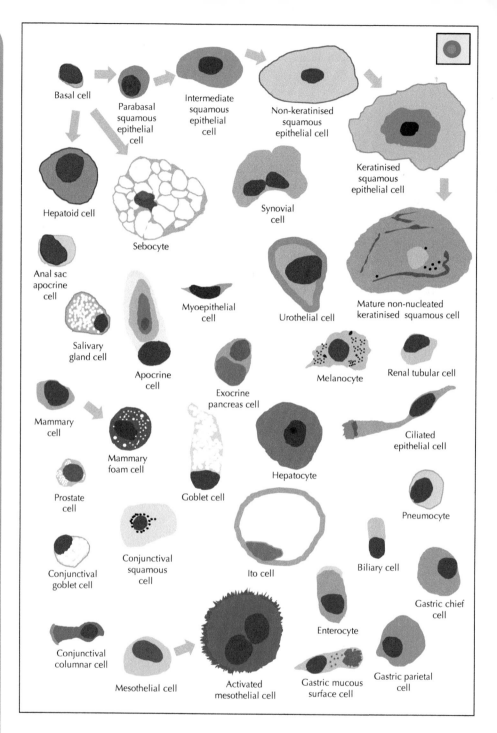

Basal cell

Parabasal squamous epithelial cell

Intermediate squamous epithelial cell

Non-keratinised squamous epithelial cell

Keratinised squamous epithelial cell

Hepatoid cell

Sebocyte

Synovial cell

Anal sac apocrine cell

Mature non-nucleated keratinised squamous cell

Salivary gland cell

Apocrine cell

Myoepithelial cell

Urothelial cell

Exocrine pancreas cell

Melanocyte

Renal tubular cell

Mammary cell

Mammary foam cell

Goblet cell

Hepatocyte

Ciliated epithelial cell

Prostate cell

Pneumocyte

Conjunctival goblet cell

Conjunctival squamous cell

Ito cell

Biliary cell

Gastric chief cell

Conjunctival columnar cell

Mesothelial cell

Activated mesothelial cell

Enterocyte

Gastric mucous surface cell

Gastric parietal cell

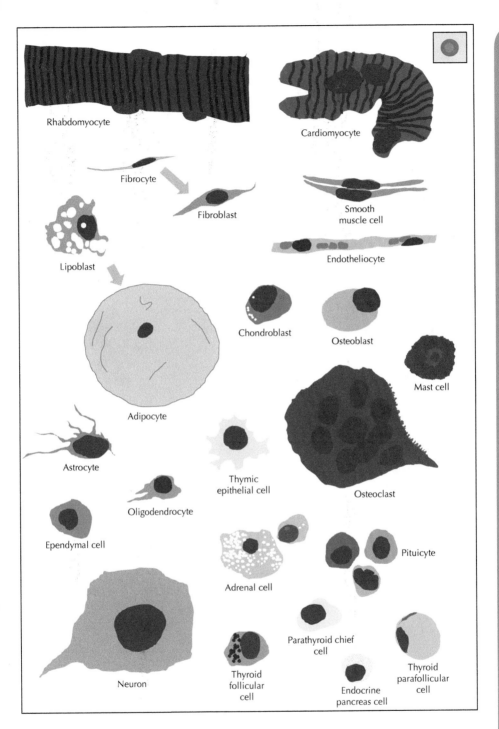

Rhabdomyocyte

Cardiomyocyte

Fibrocyte

Fibroblast

Smooth muscle cell

Lipoblast

Endotheliocyte

Chondroblast

Osteoblast

Mast cell

Adipocyte

Astrocyte

Thymic epithelial cell

Osteoclast

Oligodendrocyte

Ependymal cell

Pituicyte

Adrenal cell

Parathyroid chief cell

Neuron

Thyroid follicular cell

Endocrine pancreas cell

Thyroid parafollicular cell

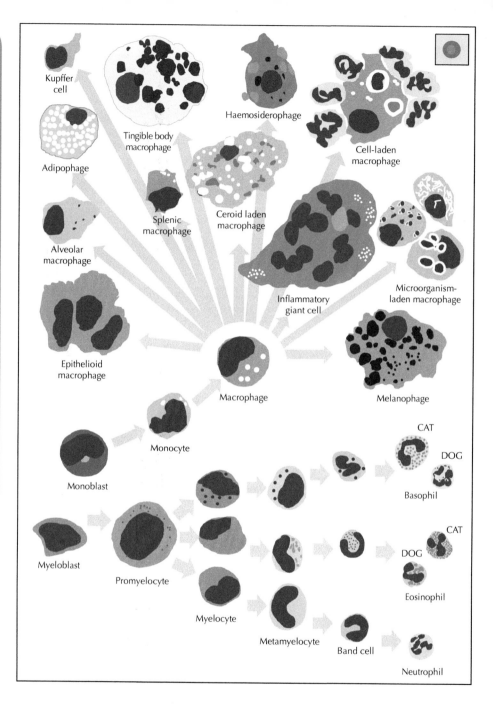

Kupffer cell

Tingible body macrophage

Haemosiderophage

Cell-laden macrophage

Adipophage

Ceroid laden macrophage

Splenic macrophage

Alveolar macrophage

Microorganism-laden macrophage

Epithelioid macrophage

Inflammatory giant cell

Macrophage

Melanophage

Monocyte

CAT

DOG

Basophil

Monoblast

CAT

Myeloblast

Promyelocyte

DOG

Eosinophil

Myelocyte

Metamyelocyte

Band cell

Neutrophil

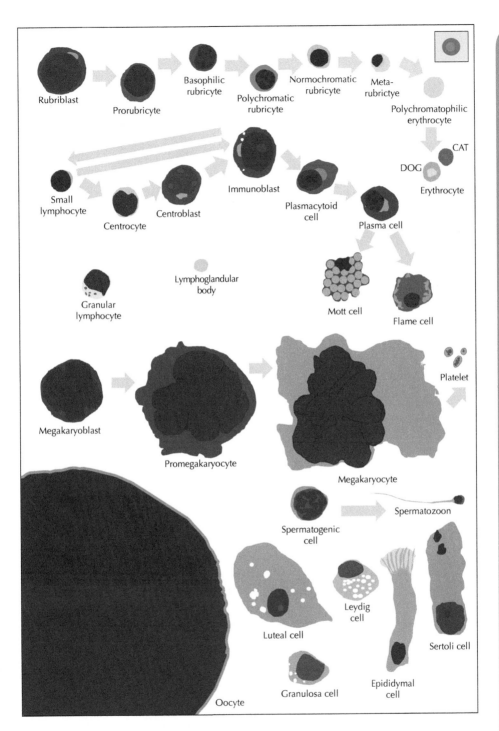

The manufacturer's authorised representative in the EU for product safety is Oxford University Press España S.A. of El Parque Empresarial San Fernando de Henares, Avenida de Castilla, 2 – 28830 Madrid (www.oup.es/en or product.safety@oup.com). OUP España S.A. also acts as importer into Spain of products made by the manufacturer.

Printed in the USA/Agawam, MA
January 13, 2025

880951.014